Praise

"Frannie O'Callaghan is like your older si[illegible]uper-cool best friend, dishing the dirt on what it's *really* like to work in a vet clinic. There's a growing body of 'vet lit,' but this is the first book I'm aware of from the vet tech's perspective, and O'Callaghan nails it. From the gross to the beautiful, from the ordinary to the extraordinary, and from the tragic to the hilarious, she covers it all with style and verve. I would consider it a must read for anyone interested in working in a veterinary clinic, or even just anyone interested in the workings of a veterinary clinic."

Dr. Philipp Schott, DVM, author of *The Accidental Veterinarian* and the Dr. Bannerman Vet Mystery series

"O'Callaghan's conversational style vignettes are raw and honest. She takes us to the back room of the vet clinic to give us an inside look at the important work veterinary technicians do, and reminds us that it's not all petting puppies and kittens. A must-read for animal lovers!"

Melinda G.McCall, DVM, author of *Driving Home Naked and Other Misadventures of a Country Veterinarian*

"A must read for anyone wishing to pursue the career path of credentialed veterinary technician. It provides a glimpse of the real day to day challenges and the dark humor we acquire from facing them. The harsh reality is we all end up a varying degree of dead inside. If you don't, you're lucky."

Kendra Dostaler, RVT, VTS (EVN)
Kendra the Vet Tech Podcast

"*SOAP Notes* is a tenacious narrative full of humor, wisdom, and compassion. Always wanted an honest, inside glimpse into the world of vet med? Here's your chance!"

Joan Gorman, RVT, MWVT Program Coordinator, American Hero VT Finalist 2016 (American Humane Society), and aforementioned Elder in the Profession

About the Author

Frannie O'Callaghan has been a licensed veterinary technician for over a decade. Apart from examining feces under a microscope, she's an avid historical fiction reader, shameless pun-user, and amateur baker. A travel nerd, she's most content hiking the Old Man of Storr during inhospitable Scottish weather, belting "Auld Lang Syne" in a Dublin pub on New Year's, or bathing with elephants in the Mae Taeng River of Thailand. Her best writing comes with heavy pours of dry prosecco. O'Callaghan lives with her husband, canine dependents, and an unfortunate number of deceased plants due to her brown thumb.

frannieocallaghan.com

SOAP Notes

FRANNIE O'CALLAGHAN

www.vineleavespress.com

SOAP Notes: Irreverent Confessions of a Veterinary Technician

Print Edition
ISBN: 978-3-98832-169-5
Published by Vine Leaves Press 2025

Cover design by Jessica Bell
Interior design by Amie McCracken
Interior illustrations by Renee Mansingh

For Jane, Dian, and Biruté, for lighting the way

Contents

Prologue 11

Welcome: Diarrhea of a Vet Tech 13
Beware of Writer 15
Definitions for the Bystanders 24
Disclaimers for the Interested Parties. 38
Location, Location, Location. 41
For the Sake of Levity: Rectal Discomfort 55

Clients: Off-Leash & Un-mange-able 57
Free Shit 59
Hoarding a Horde 70
For the Sake of Levity: Boo-Hiss. 79
For Shame 81
Inside the Joke 89
Stay Classy 92
For the Sake of Levity: To-may-to, To-mah-to 104
Bearing False Whiskers. 106
Running Interference. 122
For the Sake of Levity: Something's Afoot 129
The Lewd, The Rude, The Less-Than-Shrewd. 131

Patients: I'm Abscessed 157
Embarrassing Emergencies 159
Parvo-Land. 163
For the Sake of Levity: Shrooms & the Cathouse 173
Charity Case 1: Eggs Benedict 175
Charity Case 2: Winnie the Experiment 186
Charity Case 3: Harper 193
You Are What You Eat 197
For the Sake of Levity: Tempering Expectations 204
Love Hurts 206
Life & Death 210
For the Sake of Levity: Bears, Oh My! 219
Your Breedist Aunt 220
Know Thy Patient. 244

Professionals: Tabby, or Not Tabby 253
Know Thy Colleague 255
Emotionally Charged. 262
Drop It: Anthropomorphism in Veterinary Culture. 268
For the Sake of Levity: Anal Gland Espressos 278
Pandemic 281
Superstitious 305
Spill the Ampu-Tea. 307
Looking for Answers 314
For the Sake of Levity: Overreaction 319
What's It Take?. 321
Rewards & Compassion Fatigue 335

Epilogue 345

Author's Note

This work is a memoir of my experiences working in the veterinary field. While the recounted events are honest and true to the best of my ability, any locations, names, and identities of staff, clients, patients, and others have been altered to protect their privacy.

Illustrations are the imagined interpretations of the artist.

Prologue

Patient: *O'Callaghan, Frannie*

S: *Pf irritability and brimming with sarcasm. Other complaints include lumbar pain, degenerative patella, piss on shoes, fecal matter smeared in scrub pockets (species undetermined), dark circles under bilateral eyes, & coat unkempt. Dentition worn from grinding teeth. Ten+ years duration. Exacerbated by disorganized DVMs, snake-oil flea cures, pug nail trims, & breeder recommendations. Relieving factors include cuddling pocket-sized puppies and clients who supply coffee.*

O: *Technically adult-aged, but behavior arouses suspicion; Shoes 8.5; height 5'4"; BP: 125/80; Temp: 98.6; Weight: [*redacted, *please note 12-lb. weight-gain from breakroom donuts]*

A: *Vet tech [*see: *"burnt, out"]*

P: *Rx-1.5—3 oz. Scotch PO BID—TID. Rec. OTC NSAIDs PRN for headache and internal rage. Pt would likely benefit from home therapeutic exercises of recording written stream of consciousness. Supply with ink + paper, consider options of 80s power ballads or competitive baking shows for background noise. Allow to write uninterrupted, for 1-4 hour intervals. Force breaks for daylight, PRN.*

Welcome: Diarrhea of a Vet Tech

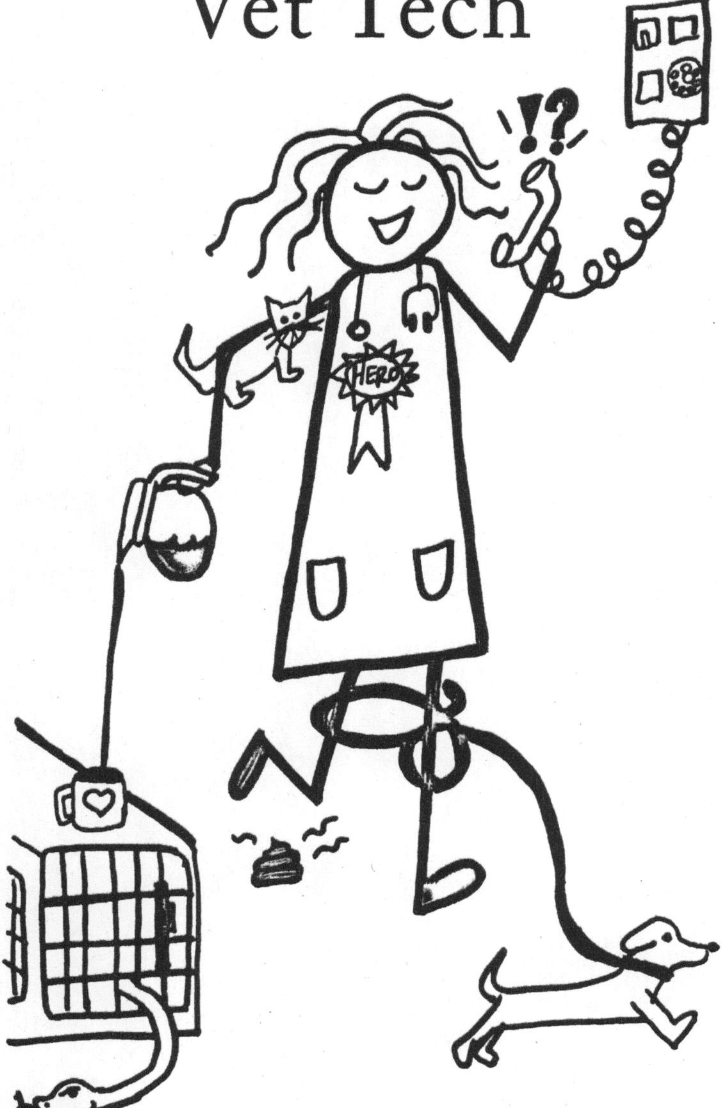

Beware of Writer

"You got to get away from words if you want to understand any animal. It thinks in pictures, it thinks in smells, it thinks in touch sensations—little sound bites like, it's a very detailed memory."
—Dr. Temple Grandin

Everything looked decent on the front page, but it was the second that mattered more. Breezing through the typical checklist of Yes and No sections on the application form, I halted at the short-answer question that usually gives me some insight into the applicant.

Why do you want to work here?

Holding my hopeful breath, I read their response,

"Because I like animals!"

I promptly exhaled in disappointment at the weak cliché. That was it? The only reason? Couldn't dig any deeper? I forced my eyes to not roll back into my skull.

No shit. Why else would anyone choose the veterinary profession?

And yet, when most young veterinary applicants get to that part, that's the immediate response. Some remember to sound a little more adult. They may spend some time coming up with craftier ways of articulating their interest. Substitute the word 'passion' for 'like' maybe. Some bullshit about connecting with the client education aspect, or a particular area of interest under the umbrella of veterinary medicine.

Not that I think their interests are bullshit. I think that anyone who's spent one, or ten, or fifty years in this insane profession had better like animals enough to stay.

I can't claim fifty years. I haven't accomplished that amount of time on Earth, yet. In the professional field, I've spent somewhere closer to the decade mark; some of those years as a newbie veterinary assistant while getting the degree that qualified me as a veterinary technician. A break while circumstances indicated veterinary job opportunities were scarce, somewhere in there. Then, after biding some time, back to it. Full-time, bona fide vet tech.

It's a hard question to answer honestly. Full confession—I don't have the perfect response crafted, either. I just know when I process those applicants, it's the overwhelming sense of their naïve optimism that makes me want to regurgitate. The clinic-based veterinary industry is considered one of the more thankless jobs according to a lot of surveys I have seen. More and more often in veterinary publications, they're cautioning our personnel about high suicide rates. Trying to offer various resources for mental health. In fact, continuing education opportunities seem to be only half-related to actually practicing medicine now, it while the rest is becoming largely dedicated to topics about stress-relief, work-life balance, and avoiding burnout. Organizational chapters now exist to combat veterinary suicides. Most of us have known someone in the field that we've lost in this tragic way. I'm saddened to count myself among them.

Sometimes it helps to go back to the beginning. To ground ourselves and remember why we started doing it in the first place. Why do we? Because … Alright, fine … we like animals.

—

On my very first day, newly employed by my first clinic, I had butterflies. Anxiety. Self-doubt. Uncertain whether I could handle the rigor of such a job. Medicine and the scientific field were a new endeavor for me, and it was daunting. Endless names of medications, unfamiliar equipment, and complicated skills on display. All those staff seemed to wield some superpower, able to move through their tasks with ease. Surely, they were so much smarter than I could ever be. It would soon be apparent how unfit I was. My hiring? A mistake.

But on that first day, I followed the veterinarian and the technician from case to case, observing how they spoke with the clients and handled the animals. Scribbling madly in a Field Notes pad carried in my scrub shirt pocket, my pen unable to keep up with the flurry of activity. What a nerd. Anyway, when they took a client's puppy to the back treatment area to complete the examination and vaccinations, they explained their process more candidly to me. The two of them stood across from each other at the exam table, with me observing and quietly absorbing their every step.

The dog was no bigger than my fist, incredibly fluffy and adorable, with a tail wagging in delight for attention. When they had determined him to be fit and healthy, the tech carefully restrained the unsuspecting puppy, while the vet administered the preventive shots. Unprepared, I jumped when the pup's high-pitched squeals of protest hit my ears, unappreciative of the first needle jab, and the one that followed. When the tech gave him a break, setting him back on the barricaded table to calm down, with no further time for consideration, the tiny patient made a beeline for me, still yelping and whimpering in offense at his treatment by the vet and tech. There was a collective 'Aww!' between the three of us as I picked him up to console him. Pleased to be the one he trusted, however undeserved, I was his safety.

In that moment, I knew I would swallow whatever feelings of inadequacy danced in my head. That I would work my ass off to do well in this job. Learn the names of those confusing drugs, figure out how the machines worked, and develop the skills to be worthy to stand alongside the other scrub-clad warriors, to hold onto that feeling of connecting with an animal.

Now, let's point out the obvious. It wouldn't be long until I would be the one having to restrain and poke patients with a needle. We learn techniques to administer them well and to reduce the amount of discomfort caused. Still, despite best efforts, sometimes the patient feels pain. We have to rise above that uncomfortable fact with the knowledge that we're treating them for the overall good of their health. That's the ultimate goal. The vet and the tech didn't do anything wrong in their handling of that tiny puppy. More times than not, my future patients would see me the same way: as the jerk who held them still, the one who administered the "torture."

We're a team of people who love animals, and that's why we're here. To improve their lives. The means of doing it can feel like a double-edged sword.

—

Why is this book titled "SOAP Notes," you ask?

No, I'm not a germaphobe who chronicles her favorite soap

brands or anything, as fascinating as that may have been. Nor is this the latest scandal-ridden veterinary-themed soap opera—although, thinking about it, I might be onto something there … Nobody take that idea, I call dibs for later! The real reason for the title is somewhat less dramatic than a long-lost-lover back from the dead yet plagued with amnesia (only to reveal he was the identical evil twin all along).

SOAP Notes refers to the acronym of a format of standard medical documentation. At least in veterinary records. Don't ask me anything about the human medical field. Gross. I wouldn't know. So. When a patient is examined at an appointment, there's a record made for every visit. S (subjective), O (objective), A (assessment), and P (plan/procedure) are the four things which ought to be present in any self-respecting patient chart.

We use tons of abbreviations I'll leave out, but otherwise? Format would look something like this:

S: What has the patient presented for? What is the problem, or purpose of the appointment? Also included in this section, client concerns and patient history. Subjective things noted on physical examination by the veterinary team. *("Presented for swollen left ear, Owner noted Patient scratching over last two weeks. Both ears have brown, waxy exudate present in ear canals. Erythematous. Caudal aspects of pinnae show self-inflicted superficial abrasions; scabbed over. Owner tried applying tea tree oil at home once, two days ago. Patient otherwise acting bright, alert, responsive. No other health concerns at this time.")*

O: Measurable items. *(Weight= 72.4 lbs / 32.9 kg, Temperature= 101.7, heart rate=85, respiratory rate=22, etc.)*

A: Diagnosis, or rule-out list of possible diagnoses. *("Otitis externa, both ears. Aural hematoma of upper half of Left pinna.")*

P: Recommended diagnostics, if any, or recommended therapies. Drugs administered, procedures done. Results seen. Follow-ups needed. Or, if the recommendations were declined, a brief description of why. *("Discussed options of surgical correction for hematoma vs. conservative treatment for OE. Due to financial constraints, Owner elects conservative treatment at this time. Ear cytology = [results]. Flushed both ears with oticetic cleanser in exam. Recommend Animax antibiotic; apply to both ears twice daily for 7-10 days. Will also send Carprofen 75 mg [7 tabs]—give 1 tablet by mouth twice daily for pain & inflammation. Recheck 10 days.")*

SOAP notes should be devoid of any emotion. It's not a diary, but a medical record. If a client hurts your feelings, that doesn't get reflected in the record. Not through sentiment. If it's relevant to the case, there's a method of recording very factually what transpired during the appointment without mentioning the client was an asshole.

Medical records are also a legal document. I make sure any VAs training with me understand that, and I'm a stickler for good notes. If it's not written in the record, it can be argued it didn't happen. In addition to this, correspondence with owners should also be documented. Any significant conversation regarding the patient, or notices pertaining to their business at the clinic should be recorded.

That comes in handy, often in very satisfying ways. I don't like to revel in another's misery, but in one case, a client called, frantic to have the dog's vaccination records emailed to a boarding facility, to where she was presently en route. She had a family emergency, needed to get out of town fast, and would be pushing it to get to the boarding drop-off before they closed for the day. I started to say, "No problem," but that quickly turned into, "Oh, well ... actually Mr. Sprinkles is technically overdue, ma'am."

I like to give people the benefit of the doubt when they're under pressure for not always acting their best selves, but that lady was ready to tear me a new asshole, because ... well, obviously this was somehow all my fault. What did I mean by that? How dare we not have informed her Mr. Sprinkles was overdue? Just, just—! She was having difficulty verbalizing her rage. With all the cheery professionalism I could muster, I read off the slew of recent attempts by our receptionists to contact her. Postcards mailed, voicemails left, email reminders ... They were on top of it. Dated and time-stamped records of attempted communications that went ignored for weeks. The lady knew she was in the wrong. I allowed her the brief despairing, "Oh, for the love of God," before she quickly changed her tune to a pleading, "What do I do?" I happened to know her designated boarding facility had onsite vets, and therefore, the capability to give vaccinations. I suggested she call ahead of her arrival to ask, nay, beg them *nicely* to please wait for her arrival and vaccinate Mr. Sprinkles.

Or, the time I got a late-evening call from a regular client, concerned she needed to urgently bring her pet in. It's never fun, but it was just one of those days where I had to tell her we were inundated and she really needed to go somewhere else. I gave two or three suggestions of nearby emergency hospitals. She didn't like that response, as she had her pet enrolled in a preventive care package with my clinic. I took great pains to explain to her that wasn't the same thing as insurance. It gave a slight discount on overall services, at best. It certainly wasn't going to cover the urgent appointment that was needed, even if we'd had time to see doggo that evening. Again, I stressed she should go elsewhere. Then I took detailed notes about the whole conversation. Which served our clinic well when she wanted to file a formal complaint later, after neglecting to take my advice about an emergency hospital. Instead, she'd waited until the dog got much worse, and then tried to make it our fault. The doctors were initially alarmed about her complaint, until they saw my documented conversation.

—

Let me be straight from the get-go. If you're reading this as some kind of spectator, curious about what veterinary staff are like, I cannot claim to represent the mindset as a whole. I'm a cynical individual with a low opinion of most people, and maybe a bit jaded. I do swear here and there, so if that offends you, this is not the reading material for you. Kindly place this book right back on the shelf or in the thrift shop donation bin where you found it.

If you're someone considering jumping into this field, whether it be starting as a kennel or veterinary assistant, think you can manage a practice, or you're one of the crazies acquiring the education to be a veterinary tech or veterinarian, good for you! But make sure you're doing it for the right reasons, have a backbone, don't mind a little blood, sweat, tears, and can still hold onto some optimism about humanity at the end of the day. Humanity, you ask? Why the fuck mention humanity, when you want to work with non-humans? Unfortunately, they come attached to the animals and will often be the biggest hurdle. As any veteran in the field will tell you, if you think your application is the gateway to playing with cute puppies and kittens all day, move along, friend. Thanks for your interest, anyway.

And finally, if you're already in the field, in one role or another, don't expect case studies here. Ain't that kind of book. Otherwise? Sláinte, mate. Some of you may see pieces of yourself in this. You may not. You may be sitting on your high horse of optimism. Figuratively, of course; I don't work with horses, as I got kicked and stomped on by them too many times. Found out during tech school that they're difficult creatures, so there went all my childhood hopes and dreams. (Spoiler, there won't be horses in this, apart from this honorable mention.) Anyways, that high horse, thinking you're a better professional than me and I have no business still being in it. Maybe. Probably. But the world is flawed, and here I still am. This writing is my own self-imposed mini-therapy session. Welcome.

Definitions for the Bystanders

"Poor planning on your part does not necessitate an emergency on mine."
—Bob Carter

What the hell is a vet tech?

Vet techs may be called by different licensing titles, depending on which state they practice in. Registered Veterinary Technician (RVT), Licensed Veterinary Technician (LVT), Certified Veterinary Technician (CVT), or even Animal Health Technician (AHT). My state uses RVT, so by habit, that will be the abbreviation used throughout this book. One holding such a title has completed an associate or a bachelor's degree of applied sciences in the field of veterinary technology. We've gone through rigorous education programs to qualify us to operate at a higher skill level in a veterinary environment.

When people ask what my job is, I usually liken it to an animal nurse, because it's the easiest description to get the point across. A lot of technicians will start bleeding out of their eyeballs, wailing, and gnashing teeth here about using this term, as they want to avoid the comparison, to be held to different titling standards from human nurses—and not that we aren't. Clearly it doesn't bother me to use "veterinary nurse" to demonstrate. Let's be honest, you see a lot of glazed-over expressions when you say, "I'm a vet tech," because the recipient of this response usually doesn't know what the fuck that is. The field of Veterinary Technology, as a recognized profession, is still relatively new. Military vet tech programs began in the 1950s, but for civilians, it took another decade.

What I *do* care about in the realm of title protection is differentiation between technician and assistant status. We'll get to the full value of the assistant role shortly, but in a nutshell? It basically comes down to education and certification. Techs have education, and assistants, on-the-job training. Trouble is, not every US state is on board (yet) with honoring that difference. That needs to happen. Rather than throwing titles around with abandon, one without educational credits shouldn't be permitted to use the correlating titling.

I digress. Whether my fellow RVTs agree with me or not on the "nurse" comparison or title protections, we can at least agree on one point. We *despise* it when we're asked, "A vet tech? Cool, so how long 'til you'll be a vet?"

Hate. Loathe. Abhor. Detest.

I don't hold it against the asker. Truly, I don't. There's a lack of understanding about what the job is, so it's an educational opportunity whenever the query is raised. Still, the question is posed so often we should start a penalty dollar-jar. We can't help that it's grating. Why? Because veterinary technology is an entirely different career path from becoming a veterinarian (DVM). Vet techs exist to support the veterinarians in their task of handling, care, and treatment of their animal patients. I like to say I know a little bit about a lot of things. A wide breadth of knowledge, but varying degrees of depth. If you're into that kind of thing, you can find any number of tacky

T-shirts with sayings about all the different job titles that RVT encompasses. *I'm a vet tech, which means I'm a: phlebotomist, radiology tech, anesthetist, surgical tech, dental hygienist, therapist, laboratory tech, pharmacy tech, restrainer/wrangler/handler, et cetera, all rolled into one.* In some nauseatingly rhyming way. And then it finishes with the corny—*What's your superpower?* Or some equally vomit-inducing cliché.

Point is, we do everything we are legally allowed to do, in practice. For a number of those things, we are often more skilled than the veterinarians. I'm good at fussy details. Taping in a venous catheter well. Identifying the subtle difference between *Trichuris vulpis* or a *Capillaria* species under the microscope. Making sure the doctor meant to say Convenia and not Cerenia, which are two entirely different injectable medications. Or Onsior versus Osurnia. (Yeah, whoever's in charge of naming drugs sometimes needs to be slapped.) Remembering to calibrate that machine and run the cleaning protocols. Predicting the behavior and appropriate handling of a stressed or volatile patient. Keeping the doctors organized, because … well, nearly all of them seem to struggle with organization in some way.

Some of us will be stronger in some skillsets than others. Some will have gone on for further certifications and specializations in an area of interest, such as behavior, dentistry, or ultrasonography. They are an even greater asset to their team, and you bet your ass, the veterinarians working alongside them rely on their judgment and knowledge.

In my state, and in most others, there are four specific things a veterinary technician cannot do. Things reserved for the veterinarians.

A veterinary technician can *not*:

- Prescribe
- Diagnose
- Perform surgery
- Administer a rabies vaccine (without supervising veterinarian's consent)

Why not? Because that's what the DVMs went to school for. Let them have their arena.

Vets spend more years and time delving into pharmacology and physiology, so they can prescribe medicine and treatments. If kitty needs an antibiotic to treat their urinary tract infection, I've got a pretty good idea of which product the doctor's going to reach for from the pharmacy shelf. However, it's not my call. I help to supply the supporting evidence—running tests, reading urinalysis results under the microscope, paying attention to the clinical signs kitty shows. Interpretation of the whole picture? I stay in my lane. Doctor makes the ultimate decision on recommended treatment.

In that same vein, neither do I diagnose. Some states go a step further to add "prognose" to the list, which is making an informed prediction of a patient's status, as far as thriving, surviving, or succumbing to a disease progression. Vets spend years longer pursuing those specific education routes. When the bloodwork results start spitting out, I may have a pretty good idea. Signs of anemia? Rises in the kidney values? Parasitic infection defense white cells? A technician should be able to recognize the main red flags, but of course it's the doctor who officially diagnoses the patient, determines whether further diagnostics are needed, and then prepares for the conversation with the owner. It's not my job to explain why the dog is in liver failure.

Performing surgery? Can't do it. Some of the older RVT generations were taught suturing, the ability to finish the skin closure, after the invasive surgery is completed by the surgeon. Some of the upcoming graduates will be, too. I was somewhere in between those generations in education, where that was left entirely to the veterinarian. It is what it is. Unless I'm closing a necropsy, I don't have the skill set to suture. Otherwise, a technician is invaluable in a surgery room. Techs help during the entire process of anesthetizing the patient; prepping the sterile surgery packs, calculating and administering drug doses, endotracheal intubation (placing the breathing tube that provides oxygen and anesthetic gas), catheter placement, running intravenous fluids, monitoring vitals during the procedure, waging war on the malfunctioning equipment and hexing it into fearful obedience again, and sometimes, they're an extra hand if the surgeon needs someone to hold some miscellaneous bit of anatomy for them. But we don't push the scalpel.

The rabies vaccine is the only legally-required vaccine for pets, which is why you can't buy that one from your local farm-supply store. An official certificate is needed as proof of administration. It's expected that it be given by a licensed vet, to ensure that it's properly done. Not that technicians can't give injections of all kinds, all day long. It's one of those technical rules most states specify. I obtain permission before I administer this particular vaccine. States often further define this rule according to a veterinary staff member's qualification. It can vary. This is what's known as Levels of Supervision. In my state, I may receive doctor permission from across the room, or even within the same building premises, whereas a veterinary assistant needs to have the veterinarian standing directly over their shoulder, watching for quality assurance.

Prescribe, diagnose, perform surgery, administer rabies vaccines. Apart from those four things, that leaves a wide berth of things RVTs *can* do.

—

The field needs good techs. They keep the practices flowing smoothly, and they excel in a role entirely separate from a veterinarian's. After first submitting my application for my VT education program, I was invited to the second phase of the process. The in-person interview. Some invaluable person gave me an insider-scoop hint prior to my appointment, which I've always remembered. If a candidate gave the instructors reason to think they were on the fence about whether they wanted to become an RVT or DVM, it was a sure way to be rejected from entry to the program. They didn't want you if you admitted to being a doctor-hopeful. And for good reason.

Speaking of the other veterinary job titles, what are they?

Let's start by establishing that every role in a clinic has value. Without all of them, the structure simply does not work as well. A good hospital has a cohesive team, but one that understands individual tasks. It's worth noting, too, no matter what your title, anyone worth a damn is willing to jump in, if they're able and needed. I'm not above cleaning a kennel if I have time to spare, and my assistant is overwhelmed. As much as I dislike it, I answer phones every day to help the front desk.

Someone once applied to my clinic seeking a receptionist role but checked the box stating they were *not* willing to deal with patient messes or handling. I rejected that application almost immediately. Good receptionists are the administrative stars we need, but I've never worked in a veterinary setting where the receptionist wasn't needed to get their hands dirty alongside the rest of us. Pretty much on the daily.

I worked as a relief tech once in a hospital, covering odd shifts here and there. The receptionist was a guy who got to know me well enough to learn I hated being at the front desk. Nonetheless, I noticed one afternoon on the security cameras a line of clients, all at once. Didn't want to, but I went to his aid. Filled a script for someone waiting. Got the client checked out and on their way. By then, the queue was already under control. Nothing strenuous. A daily task. Still, he took it upon himself to create and print up a silly "Hero of the Day" certificate dedicated to me, with some descriptive blurb about conquering my hatred of the 'hazardous territory' of the reception. Little things, y'all. Took only a few minutes to help a friend.

By now, we've already touched on most of the jobs, but let's consolidate.

Kennel Assistant or *Kennel Technician*. Usually in charge of walking boarding dogs, feeding patients and/or boarders, cleaning kennels, and other hospital maintenance. This is usually considered the most unskilled position and often relegated to young staff members just getting their foot in the door. Or part-time high school or college kids. Even so, you need someone intuitive or experienced with animals. Wary of safe practices. Able to spot when something may be wrong. Whenever I help to hire someone, I look for detail-oriented people. Observant people. They're harder to find than you would think.

Veterinary Assistant. There may be some crossover with both the kennel assistant and the tech. An assistant has no veterinary-specific education or certification. They have on-the-job training and are expected to be less skilled than a technician. Which is not to say I haven't met assistants who know their shit or have years of experience on me. Ones who have earned their right to a fair amount of respect for their knowledge. They handle many similar tasks as the RVTs, but usually at an entry skill level. My current assistants can look at a fecal sample with me and are improving at spotting a parasite egg under the microscope, for example. However, they usually need help with the species identification, couldn't tell you much about the concerns or origin of that parasite without looking it up, and would probably need to consult my reference charts for the appropriate dewormer. They haven't followed an entire course in parasitology, as a tech does. Of course, the longer they spend on the job applying themselves to the subject, the more they'll pick up. Again, some VAs may do the job very well, but they aren't expected to have studied the material in the same depth as an RVT.

Registered Veterinary Technician. Has educational credits. See previous answer.

Groomer. A groomer may or may not be present in a veterinary hospital. They know their stuff and I could never do their job. I don't have the patience for that brand of fuss. I could never trim a neat fringe on a Schnauzer or listen to huskies whine at me in the bathtub nonstop. Everything would go home looking as bad as my crooked bangs in my third-grade school photo. Best I can do is an even medical groom, and no stylist will boast about it. (A medical groom entails shaving fur for clinical treatment, whether for a dermatological issue, wound, or in preparation for a surgical field.) Many groomers are adept at spotting when something is concerning and recognizing the need to consult the medical team's advice.

A hidden tumor under the fur or raging ear infection, for example. Sometimes, God forbid, they accidentally nick or lacerate delicate skin and then seek us for the assist. Human beauticians probably don't have to deal with their clients being jumpy or biting. Or anal glands.

Receptionist. This seems a pretty obvious role, but they're often the unsung heroes in the hospital. The face that greets clients. Approachable and caring, but effective. We rely on them to not only answer the phones, order supplies, schedule appointments and staff shifts, handle billing, and discharge instructions, but to have a basic knowledge of how veterinary procedures will best flow for the team. They are the first line of triage and prioritize what is of highest medical concern. Now, I still have to explain to my receptionist the difference between a histopathology or a cytology test every time, so she knows how to charge the client appropriately. That's fine. She didn't go to school for it, and I won't bore her with the minutiae. That said, for an endless number of medical scenarios, she knows what urgent questions to ask clients over the phone, to decide if a patient is potentially blocked, for example, or if the risk of foreign body obstruction is there.

Office Manager. This person may have duties which cross over with the receptionist. Or a clinic owner. They may handle financial decisions and personnel matters. Possibly some marketing stuff. Vital face and leadership role.

Veterinarian. Remember the four things I said an RVT couldn't do? That's the very generalized list of what a Doctor of Veterinary Medicine (DVM) does. They spend years in school (with corresponding debt) to be able to treat animals. There's a tired joke out there that goes something like,

"What happens when veterinarians fail out of school?"

—Dunno. What?

"They become doctors instead!"

The point is, similar to vet techs having an abundance of knowledge over a wide array of subject matter, veterinary doctors are asked to be the go-to for every aspect of an animal's well-being and health. Not only that, but for several species, rather than just one. For your *Homo sapiens* medical needs, if you have a foot problem, you go to your podiatrist. Heart problem, cardiologist. Knee pain, you go to … you get it. For animals? Veterinarians do it all.

As mentioned, a tech's main objective is to support their veterinarians in the individual cases seen. For my formative learning years, I adhered pretty strictly to that, well aware I was learning. One of the things I learned quickly was to adapt to different doctors' styles of medicine. Not everyone has the same approach. Some may be quite by-the-book, and others are willing to go off-roading. Some prefer to offer everything under the sun for gold standards, whereas others suggest a more conservative approach. Or straight-shooters versus the impassioned bedside manner. I might prefer one method over another, but nine times out of ten, I have respect for all the theories behind the methods. There's not necessarily a right or wrong way to do things. Sometimes one philosophy is a better fit for a particular client, for instance. It's my job to assist, either way.

I used to work with a by-the-book doctor at a big facility. One day I hesitated before grabbing the ear cleansing solution for her patient, trying to remember which one to select from the basket of options. With her keen eye for detail, Dr. A homed in on that moment of delay, taking the time to explain to me exactly why she preferred the cleansing option that she did. Why it was the best technique. The perfect antimicrobial dilution. At the end of the mini lecture, Dr. A was looking for affirmation that I agreed with her logic and would swear by it.

I had to disappoint her, reminding her of my role.

"Dr. A, I'm perfectly happy to use your method when I'm helping with your patient, but ... you know when I'm working Dr. B's patient, I have to do it his way. Or with Dr. C's patient, then I have to choose her ear cleanser."

Dr. A pursed her lips, clearly still having an opinion on her superior method, but she suppressed whatever comments were swirling in her head.

Years later, when I started my longest-term position, I met one of the veterinarians I would be working with. Serving as the only technician in a small clinic, I wanted to make a good first impression. Right off the bat, she asked me what my style was. How I preferred to do things.

I was taken aback.

Why did that matter? I was accustomed to tailoring my work to whichever veterinarian I worked under. It was her opinion that was relevant. Not mine.

I said as much in response. That I was flexible and would do things the way she preferred. Taking her cues.

She pushed back, insisting I be permitted some freedom of shared expertise.

A few years in, I sometimes wonder if she regretted that. Indeed, I got comfortable. Because I was the only tech in that clinic, I had quite a bit of freedom to set things up the way I liked. She and I had a decent system of working together. A flow to the rhythm of our surgery routines or room appointments. I'm sure I grated on her nerves for the strong opinions

I developed, but it was a two-way street. And we usually had a sense of humor about it. Throwing flack back and forth about stylistic choices. I tended to err on sizing up for IV catheters, but down on endotracheal tubes, whereas she was the opposite, for example.

"Psh, you chose that baby catheter for me? Come on. He can handle a twenty-gauge."

Yet even as I threw her twenty-two-gauge catheter back in the drawer in favor of the larger size, I appreciated working alongside a good veterinarian who gave me space to have my opinions. To succeed in areas of my skill. By the same token, she had my respect. I trusted her judgments on a case and did my best to perform the work in such a way that made her work easier. It all came back to the service of the patient, and I didn't take for granted that our good teamwork aided the mission.

She became a good friend. That's not required, as long as you can get along with your team. But it helps. We talked about personal stresses, latest good reads, and any small-town drama. She's the cuddler of the patients. Generous enough to host a fun gathering of staff. The kind of person who would handle your disastrously flooded basement while house-sitting for you, swearing 'it's not that bad!' and to just enjoy your vacation.

As an aside, the veterinarian/owner who hired me for this position conducted his interview over the phone. All within the same call from the clinic, inquiring whether I was still interested since applying. I'd been about to order ice cream from a drive-thru when the phone rang and had to pull over in the parking lot. Trying to stay calm about answering the questions. With my resumé to peruse, he went through some of the general items about my education and such. Confirmation of the necessary veterinary details. But that didn't interest him as much as another brief mention in my employment history. He remarked about the bartending shifts I'd been working while I was between veterinary gigs.

"So," he said. "How would you make me an Old Fashioned?"

Quickly, I had to revert my brain from vet med-themed tangents I could go on, and instead, mentally put myself behind the bar with a beer-soaked towel slung over my shoulder.

"Well, you'd want to start by selecting your whiskey first. Typically, a bourbon," I began, and then added descriptive details of each step, mainly to stall while I tried not to panic-forget the difference between that libation and my preferred Manhattan, which is a similar recipe. Thankfully, I got the remaining ingredients of bitters and simple syrup correct. (Manhattan uses sweet Vermouth in place of syrup.) I wasn't sure if he was testing whether I was lying about that particular credential, had worth as a bartender, or just hoped I could mix him up a drink after a long day, if hired.

Regardless, it worked out. Knowing how to make an Old Fashioned off the top of my head helped me to get my vet tech job. He had few to no other questions for my interview. We don't drink on the clock, (duh) but I will say I earned my spot as the go-to cocktail shaker for any office party.

I should probably put some kind of obvious disclaimer that this was an unconventional interview question, and not to be expected for most RVTs in the job-searching phase.

DISCLAIMER: *RVTs are not required to moonlight as drink-slingers, or even to like alcohol, but hey, it can't hurt to have a classic cocktail recipe memorized. You never know.*

There.

Personally, I love creativity questions. Maybe that was part of what attracted me to working in this location. When I conduct an interview, I throw one in. Not necessarily about booze, but something that requires half an imagination. Tells me something about how the candidate thinks on their feet. In this case, it told me something about the person hiring me for the job. That was an insight that I think turned out to be right. Not that we don't butt heads occasionally, too, but he's been a good boss. The generous kind of guy who hands you a few extra crisp bills before you jet off to take advantage of your vacation hours, with instructions to spend it unwisely. Or on the hottest day in summer, he's the guy who personally helps move a spare refrigerator into your home, when your old one kicked the bucket.

Working with good people matters. Choose well.

Disclaimers for the Interested Parties

"You cannot get through a single day without having an impact on the world around you. What you do makes a difference, and you have to decide what kind of difference you want to make."
—Dr. Jane Goodall

It bears repeating. If you think you want to be in the field to pet cute puppies and kittens all day—don't. It's what we like to promote, but that perception is just our Instagram filter. Not the reality of the job.

While cute animals do happen, it's icing on the cake. A urine, pus, blood, anal gland, vomit, shit-filled cake. Frequently, patients coming to see me must be dragged through the front door. They're utterly terrified. We do our best to win them over, but it's a simple fact that most don't want anything to do with us. Especially if they're already injured or sick. Many of them will act aggressively towards us. No matter what the root cause of their aggression is, we have to figure out how to safely restrain the animal with sharp teeth and claws.

You have to want this: the chance to improve the welfare of animals.

There will be hair. A lot of it. Invest in lint rollers. There will be scars. There will be piss in shoes and shit in pockets. No, really. I had a record week once where I got peed on before 9:00 a.m. every single day. It's amazing how often I carry a nervous patient from point A to point B, only to later realize they dropped a sneaky fecal-bomb into my scrub pocket. Or like that time in tech school when we had a rat lab class. Friendly little patients, and fun to handle. The following week, we moved on to the next species. My classmate was listening to the lecture on guinea pigs while idly playing with the piece of "trash" left behind in her lab coat pocket. Only to finally pull it out to examine it, and realize it wasn't the gum wrapper she thought, but yeah. Rat shit.

Personal space goes away. We encounter all kinds of weird medical scenarios. We'll talk to clients about their pets humping teddy bears too much, with a serious face. We'll pull animal hair splinters out of our skin. We'll find ourselves in compromisingly close positions with coworkers just to safely restrain a patient. Crotch-sniffing dogs will announce to the whole exam room when we're menstruating. If we (humans) ever have a private medical issue of our own, sometimes clever vets may see if they can't puzzle it out based on our symptoms … and they're usually right.

And if you're thinking you might get into it for the money? Ha … hahaha … hahahaha!

Let's move on.

No … really. Let's move o—Ok, ok, fine.

No, you're not gonna get rich being a vet tech. You'll never hear any vet tech say, "Hey, look into this job, the money's great!"

If we've stuck it out in the veterinary field, it's because we have a passion for animals or the science in some form or another. Nobody's here for any boastful paycheck. I could get a desk job with probably significantly less headache, poop, urine, blood, teeth, and claws and be far better paid to do it. Instead, I've stayed in a position that asks for a pretty high level of skill for relatively poor income. If you're considering this field, search online for expected salaries in your own area or intended area. Some facilities will offer better pay than others, of course, depending on their office culture and location. By office culture I mean how well they value a technician. Not all clinics or hospitals treat technicians the same. If there's no differentiation between a tech and an assistant role, it's not the best place for you. If a technician is appreciated, another factor to consider includes affordability of the neighborhood. Usually, we can get by with modest living. I have yet to meet any independently-wealthy cohort in the field.

Now can we stop talking about money?

Location, Location, Location

"In business, wrong location leads to suffocation."
—Mokokoma Mokhonoana

Still here? Fine.

The veterinary field is starved for good help. If you're desperate to get your foot in the door, that's good news for you. Some flexibility with location may be required, but let's talk about that prime rule of real estate.

Big city, small town, or country vet? As far as clinical practice is concerned, I've had the experience of working in all three settings in the Midwest. There's no right or wrong answer to selecting any of these places over another. It all comes down to individual preference. Do you like the adrenaline of a faster pace, or prefer a calmer environment to handle cases? Does the practice incite competition between the doctors on staff, or does it promote positive team energy? Private practice or corporate? Have you considered the clientele, and their expectations, needs, and budgets? Every kind of person keeps pets. All clinics deal with a variety of owners, regardless. But the location of a practice dictates an overall trend in the type of clientele it usually experiences. Are they paying you what you're worth, with respect to your experience and education? What's the mindset of the place? The vibe? The motto?

If you're in the veterinary field, chances are good you have options for employment. If the culture of one place isn't working for you, find another.

Culture matters. What you surround yourself with matters.

When I first left home for college, I had a few friends from high school I could lean on for support. Familiar faces to help with the transition to a new place. Somewhere around Junior year, I changed my mind about my major and left to take on this idea of Veterinary Technology. My university didn't have any such program, and I had to find a community college nearby that did. I went solo. Quite literally, I sobbed while driving myself and my possessions in a packed car away from all the friends I'd made over the previous university years. Yes, it probably looked as pathetic as it sounds. My first time having an apartment completely alone, starting a new job, and going to a school where I truly knew no one. I spent three years working in that major city, living paycheck to paycheck while attending vet tech school.

It was the first and only corporate clinic I've worked in. I loved my team. Adored my team. I wouldn't say I'm terribly shy. I talk when I want to. Engage when I want to. But I'm most definitely an introvert. With new life circumstances and being terrified of my job for the first three or four months, it was hard not to form an emotional bond to the doctors, receptionists, veterinary technicians, and assistants I saw almost every day.

After being in my newly chosen field for all of three-ish weeks, still feeling like a fish out of water, I had a shit day. Another morning when I drove to the job, the weight of fearful anticipation was heavy in my gut. When I arrived, things kept going wrong. I spilled a bottle of pyrantel dewormer all over the counter. Assisted with a patient blood draw that went poorly. And while still trying to learn the complicated array of vaccines available in the fridge, I'd spent a huge amount of time painstakingly comparing each vial to the patient record I was preparing for. Double-checking the notes. Triple-checking the vial labels to see that they matched. Making sure I drew up the correct vaccinations, pyrantel dose, heartworm test, and fecal kit for the upcoming appointment, only to realize one of the experienced coworkers had already prepared that patient's tray. I'd wasted both time and effort unnecessarily.

The final straw that day was when I popped blood samples into the centrifuge to be spun down, as I had several times before. Clicked the lid into place and hit the start button. Seconds later, there was shattering POP! Followed by a flash of light and awful machine grinding noises. Everyone in the vicinity jumped in alarm.

Gawking at the smoking machine, I was horrified when the hospital director opened the lid to reveal the explosion. Broken parts of machinery, strewn everywhere. Collection tubes, distorted, and blood smears painting the walls of the centrifuge. Some kind of electric short circuit. It wasn't my fault, but at that moment, it didn't matter. As the button-presser, I felt responsible. Emotion was quickly welling to the surface. I broke the machine that cost God-knew-how-much, and would probably have to pay for it from my poor student's bank account, and it was surely the worst fate in the world to have to collect a new sample from the patient.

Before the tears even had a chance to make their way out, I felt someone slam into the back of me. One of my new coworkers. A head shorter than me and with a smaller frame, but the most confident tech I've ever met. If she'd been bigger, she might have knocked me over. She wrapped her arms around my waist and bear-hugged me tightly. No hesitation, no questions asked. Forcing comfort when it was needed.

"It's ok," she said firmly. "It's not your fault. You're ok!"

Her reassurances didn't stop me from bursting into tears. Still, due credit for her considerate and swift response. I was eventually able to pull myself out of my ass, calm down, and regroup. It helped that the Chief of Staff thought the incident was funny (though he was under stern orders not to laugh in front of me while I was still crying), and no one expected me to replace the centrifuge. Everyone promised me it was no big deal to get another sample from the patient.

It felt like a self-imposed initiation, though. A turning point. I'd embarrassed myself in front of everyone, cried at work, and had a shitty day. The team had had my back. I knew it was ok to go back the next day. And the day after. Surely it couldn't get worse than that.

Ha, of course it's gotten worse than that! This is veterinary medicine. Still, I survived my first shit day, and that meant I could do it again. Having a good group of people at your side makes all the difference during the bad days.

Incredible team aside? I have nothing nice to say about the corporate monster. I'll never do that again. In a corporate hospital, a bunch of upper-level administrators can come to your clinic and find things to correct about a place they don't work in, day-to-day. If a practice model worked well for a clinic in Albuquerque, well, then they decide they should mandate that model across the board. The clinics in Cincinnati and Milwaukee and St. Louis should do the same. Never mind their own systems.

They'd tell us, of course, they respected us in our roles as technicians (or whatever), and no one was expected to be a salesman. Yet they turned around and rated our job performances every quarter on how many preventive care packages we sold to clients. How many new enrollments had my name attached to the case. If I didn't convince clients, why not? I didn't go to vet tech school, nor work my ass off to earn the degree so I could be a fucking salesman. If my performance review is based on that data, call a spade a damn spade. Those reviews also rated us according to how well we fulfilled expectations. *Below*, *Meeting*, or *Exceeding Expectations* were the options. Usually I was lucky enough to be in the "Meeting" category. One of the technicians I looked up to was, more than once, considered "Below." If one was "Exceeding," well, then, they might have grounds to ask for a raise, and that's not where the business wanted us.

Oh, and the competition thing? If my previous phrasing wasn't a dead giveaway, that shit pissed me off. Working in a clinic, it should be a team. Helping each other. Feeling able to count on folks to fulfill their title roles and wanting to do your own part. For the good of our patients. That's the whole point. Our corporate overlords liked to push incentives that made our doctors compete against each other to win over the most clients. There is value in continuity in some medical cases, but you won't convince me those administrators gave a fuck about that. Even the rest of the team were expected to help facilitate the game. The pressure to finish appointments that way? Tacky as hell.

"Did you have a good experience with Dr. Such-and-Such today?"

"Yeah, it was fine, I gu—?"

"Great, let's make sure they're your Primary Provider from now on. I've marked it on your account!"

Brownie performance points for Dr. Such-and-Such. Again, I loved all the doctors I worked with, but I was deliriously happy when we finally got rid of that fucking incentive. It pitted them against each other. If a client did best with a particular vet, they usually told us their preference anyways when they made an appointment, and we had the option of assigning them without needing it to be forced down our throats by a party that shouldn't have been involved in the decision. Most clients felt uncomfortable when we asked.

Alright, enough about corporate. Back to the point at hand.

Big City Clinics.

The obvious takeaway was the fast pace and high volume of cases seen. Not much time for idleness. My clinic was one of the few in its neighborhood open on Sundays. My boss was not opposed when I deemed them *Bloody Sundays*, for the complete disregard for going beyond case capacity. That aside, it came down to money and mindset. Pardon the mass generalization, because there are always exceptions, but most city owners could afford a higher level of care for their pets. Whether or not they were *willing* to spend money is another matter altogether. But it is true that, if Fido needed expensive diagnostics or involved procedures, and the client trusted your recommendation, they were more likely to go for it than in other areas. They expected that quality of care.

Every clinic has at least one client who's a cat hoarder. (I currently have a handful, at least.) Whenever we called to tell ours what treatment we thought was important for Fluffy Number 19, our cat-hoarding client there would consistently tell us, "Whatever s/he needs is fine, you know you don't need to ask." Well, we did still need to ask. We never wanted to take advantage and assume. But that lady would rather go bankrupt than deprive one of the cats of medical need. Another client was fond of reminding us which airplane hangar he owned at the major airport, before exclaiming how low our prices were compared to clinics on the coast.

I always went into an exam room with a proposed treatment plan that was considered the Gold Standard of care. It didn't matter who you were. If Dr. What's-Their-Face thought a pet needed radiographs, bloodwork, an ultrasound, this procedure, or those expensive medications, it was my job to show the top-of-the-line recommendation. Many would simply say "Go for it." Not that we judged harshly when someone operated within a budget. It happened plenty. But they were still shown that estimate first. Then we whittled it down from there, to what they could afford to give for care for their pet.

The drawback to the city clients? There's a profound lack of common sense, I have to say. Not that they didn't usually have good intentions, but while obtaining a patient history, I often bit my tongue about the idiotic things I heard. I'm not qualified to say this with certainty, but my suspicion is that over recent generations, humans have gotten further away from the natural world. We don't live among nature nearly as much as we used to. Most of us, especially in cities and suburbs, have many degrees of separation from fields, woods, ponds, rivers, wild animals, and the like. I think with that observation missing, some people have little awareness of how any of it works. I guess this is my SOAPBOX moment to say, go on more nature hikes.

Country Clinics.

My stint in a country clinic was admittedly rather short. It wasn't a good fit for me. That doesn't mean it's not great for the next person, but if I ever have to hear another country song about girls in short jorts or old farm trucks on a dusty road, I may do something violent. The five staff each got to choose the Pandora radio station one day of the week, and friends, my Tuesdays were the *only* days the clinic didn't listen to honky-tonk hymns. I can recall a euthanasia appointment on one of my radio days. I know what's professional and what's not, and there was nothing on my station that could have been called inappropriate. Turning the volume down would have been fine, but I'll never forget the veterinarian turned the station back to country music during that euthanasia appointment, *just in case* the client may have found it off-putting to hear anything else.

You may think I'm joking, but if you despise the music selection, it's enough to drive you mad. For the record, I have every respect for the classic country greats like Johnny Cash or Patsy Cline. That wasn't what I got. The newer hillbilly crap isn't my cup of tea.

There ended up being a laundry list of reasons why I didn't stay more than a few months at that location. Besides a long commute, strong differences of opinion on the quality of care were a problem, and I had to stand up for myself in that regard. Lack of that team-spirit vibe I'd been so lucky to have at the other place. I was sure the one other technician didn't like me. Other staff were distant. My favorite coworker was a receptionist, and we didn't have much cause to spend significant time around each other. I didn't mind a slow-down of pace after the madness of the city, but many days were so slow I was bored out of my mind. One can only scrub the barn from top to bottom so many times. The large animal crew had more to do, but I wasn't usually their pick for those runs. I'd spent most of my time learning small animal medicine. I knew my large animal knowledge was weak, and I'd been upfront about it. I never got the guidance there I was hoping for. Maybe that's just a cultural thing I'm not used to. Getting thrown in, to sink or swim. I'm ok with an intentional challenge. In this case, it read not as a challenge presented to help me improve, but complete indifference.

I was depressed there and made the decision it wasn't working.

What will I say for it? (And remember, I'm massively generalizing.) The clients were good people. I also came to expect the reverse of city culture. In the country, while people were *not* as willing to put much money into an animal that was just a pet (livestock is another story, and I won't get into that), they were not lacking in common sense. Instead, when I obtained my patient history there, I usually found myself thinking, "Oh, they tried X after Y symptom occurred? That was smart."

It was also probably one of the nicer facilities I've worked at. Perhaps that's unexpected of a country clinic, but that practice owner went for as much state-of-the-art equipment, bells and whistles as he could. Aesthetics were important to him, and the place looked sleek.

Actually, there was a day one of the VAs was asked to fertilize the perfectly-manicured grass around the building. I'm not a fucking landscaper. Neither was this VA. I don't know what the hell he did but he clearly used the wrong product by mistake and ended up *killing* all the grass instead. I shouldn't have laughed, but it was something to drive to work every day and see the recently golf-worthy green disintegrated to brown twigs. Don't worry, the kid didn't get fired. He worked his ass off, performing the manual labor to replace the new grass patches when they arrived. Some thousand-odd dollars of damage. The grass isn't especially relevant, except that it's important to have a sense of humor about things. Oh, and to work hard to fix it when you fuck up.

Small Town Clinics.

The small town was where I resided and practiced the longest. I don't have to get too deep into the woods to say that culturally, it was a good balance of the previous two. The pace was manageable. I wasn't usually twiddling my thumbs with boredom, but nor did I go home overwhelmed and exhausted. My Goldilocks sweet spot. I got a wider variety of everything there. Kept it interesting. I had clients willing and able to be big spenders, but they were vastly outweighed by the ones struggling to afford monthly flea and tick prevention. Still, the overall majority were somewhere in-between. The reasonable, everyday folks.

If one was in financially-strapped circumstances, we usually had no problem trying to work with them, to give appropriate care within their budget. If they were a proven client, we helped to figure out some payment plan. It was only when people were deceptive, such as waiting until the checkout point of the appointment to say, "Oh, I don't get paid until next Friday," that we got upset. Which happened frequently. We were burned enough that we could no longer offer those options to new clients. There are surely plenty of honest people out there who mean it when they ask if they can make partial payments. They got upset when we had to say no. I felt for them, but the few ruined it for the majority.

Overall, it was a reasonable, down-to-earth place to be. Which was not something to take for granted. Being able to relate to the clients whose animals you cared for was paramount. Folks often asked, "What would you do, if it was your pet?" in any given circumstance. With the caveat that it wasn't my place to make the decision for them, I worked in an environment where I felt comfortable giving an honest opinion. There's not always a black-and-white answer to the dilemma, and I'd gotten decent at asking guided questions. A small-town clinic didn't pressure staff to push for unnecessary treatments. They didn't recommend expensive care if they didn't feel it would deliver a worthwhile outcome for the pet. We were willing to have a straightforward conversation about what worked for the owner. About all of it, budget, prognosis, or implementation of recommended treatment.

It wasn't glamorous, but it was my happy place. Still, to each their own.

The Honorable Mention.

I can't finish this chapter without discussion of the most horrific interview I've ever been to. I've tried to stress the importance of being proud of the place you work. If you walk into a building and your first thought is, "Oh, I can fix that up …" that's a problem.

Don't ignore the red flags.

This clinic was a very, very small-town facility that I interviewed with before graduating from tech school, preparing to move in with my then-fiancé, to another town. I'm a proponent of trying new experiences, but I admit I was slapped in the face with culture shock at this location. Still working in my Big City clinic at the time, I was accustomed to the importance of peak professionalism. When I first arranged the interview over the phone, the veterinarian informed me it was a casual process, and I could come and observe operations on the given afternoon. I asked him if he preferred that I wear scrubs to the interview.

"Ma'am, I don't care if you show up in a bikini," he drawled. (Red flag.)

I didn't, by the way.

But I did go and was subsequently taken aback to walk into the clinic with concerningly outdated décor, peeling wallpaper, and just ... filth. Layers of dirt. There were literal stacks of paper, medical records, and cardboard boxes nearly reaching the ceiling. (Red fl ... you know what, you can spot them yourself from now on. I believe in you.) How they ever found any files was beyond me. The veterinarian/owner refused to hire a receptionist. He felt they were a waste of time, only occupied with such things as sitting around painting their nails, on his dime. I wish I was making that up. I'm not. I could have thought of a few good reasons to hire a receptionist when I observed his poor fucking technician, unable to do her job properly.

I wondered if she knew it wasn't normal to stop working on a dental patient under anesthesia, leaving them *still intubated and unattended* in a cage, while she had to run to answer the door or phone. You know, things a receptionist could handle when she was done painting her nails. If you're not in the field and at all unsure, it is never ok to leave an anesthetized patient alone that way, especially still with an endotracheal tube in place. Never ever. That's 101. But that's what the asshole of a vet allowed, because he wouldn't properly staff his facility.

I stayed with the neglected patient while she answered the front door.

Next, I had the misfortune of seeing a radiography process. They wheeled out a decades-old, yellowing machine. Prepared their patient in the proper position. As no one had offered me any protective lead shields, I cooperatively stepped outside of the room for safety's sake. God knew what kind of scatter radiation that thing emitted.

The veterinarian proceeded to laugh at me.

He assured me it was no big deal. They used that machine all the time without any kind of protective shield. And hey, his formerly-pregnant employee used to take X-rays for him all the time without any, and her kid turned out fine!

If I wasn't horrified already at the complete disregard for anesthetic safety protocols, this was a new level. Just a big middle finger to every OSHA standard regarding radiology. His employees should have sued. What's sadder is they probably had no idea.

I couldn't tell you why I didn't just run out of the building screaming then, as seemed fitting. I stayed long enough to witness appalling etiquette with his clients. Not bothering to even pretend he knew anything about the patients that showed up in his exam room. No patient charts. No pleasantries. No bedside manner. It was clear the large animal operation was his breadwinner. I'd say if you brought a cow to him, it would probably be fine. But any small animal ought to have joined me in running for the hills. Putting as much distance between them as possible.

There was no sit-down formal Q-and-A or anything of that nature. I eventually found an excuse to leave. He didn't ask me when I could start, nor did I ask when I might hear back. It was probably mutual: I wasn't what he was looking for, and I wanted no part of him.

There are horrors out there. Of course, most clinics don't deserve to wear a perpetual cone of shame. Don't lose sight of good standards of medicine but be open to different practicing styles and cultures.

Wear a fucking lead apron in the radiology room, for starters.

For the Sake of Levity: Rectal Discomfort

It's crucial to have a sense of humor when you work in a medical field. Veterinary medicine is no exception. And if it's a little crude sometimes, even better. Because things can get messy. You have to roll with the punches.

The first moment of levity I'll share was one such rude occasion.

Dog with a rectal mass presented to recheck the progressive growth. The owner had opted out of taking his pet to any specialist, so we were seeing him on the terms of keeping the dog comfortable and making sure bodily functions could still occur properly for his final days. I had the onerous task of restraining the unhappy canine while the veterinarian did his rectal exam. As you can imagine, it was painful for the dog, and though we kept it as brief as possible, the affair involved a bloody mess in a sensitive location. All over the vet's gloved hand, running down the dog's legs, and dribbling heavily onto the exam table.

Fast forward a few minutes later, after clean-up. While I counted the refill of Prednisone pills to send home with the owner, the veterinarian came in beside me at our pharmacy station.

"Boy," he said with a deadpan tone. "I really tore that dog a new asshole."

Focused on my counting, I gave it a polite chuckle in the moment. But later that night, I kept thinking about it, and each time, progressively laughing a little more. A little harder.

Years later, the one-liner still gives me giggle fits.

Clients: Off-Leash & Un-mange-able

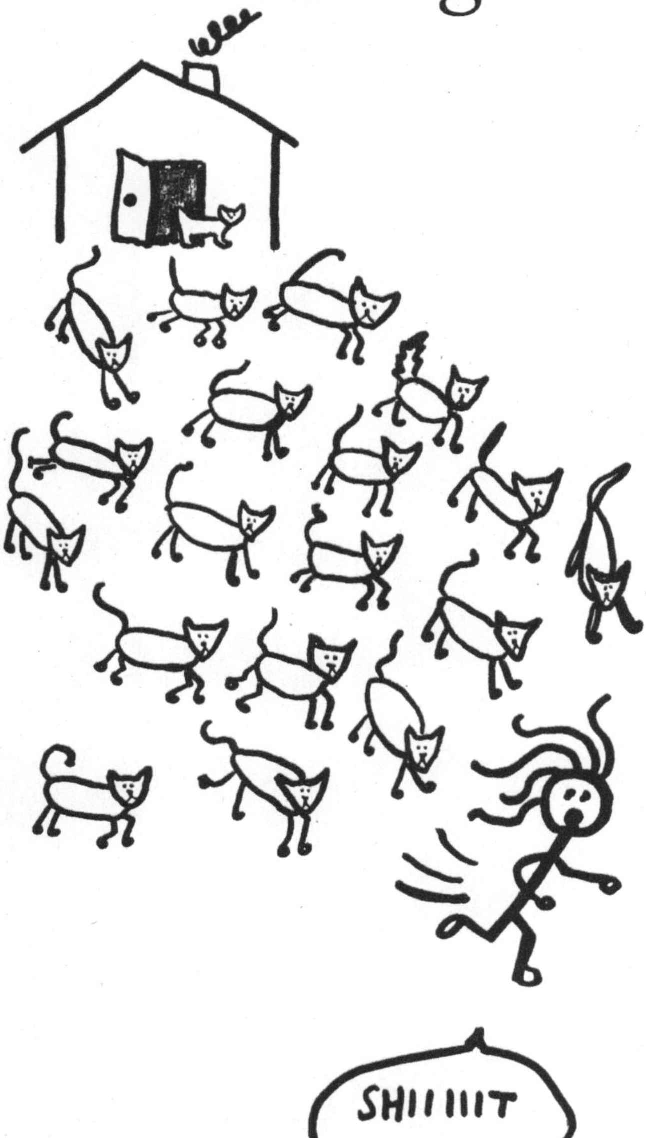

Free Shit

"If you're good at something, never do it for free."
—Joker, from *The Dark Knight Rises*

If you enter the veterinary profession, I can make you one specific guarantee, no matter your role within the hospital setting. So, what great declaration can I make with such confidence? Here it is.

Your friends will ask you for free animal advice.

Don't get me wrong. If we're good friends, I don't mind lending my professional opinion about your pet. Maybe there's a time when I could use advice from your own area of expertise. I know I've made those inquiring calls, too. It's a nice courtesy, as long as it's reciprocal.

But like most nice things, it gets easily abused. There are certain names saved in my phone that, when I see them flash on my home-screen, my immediate reaction is, "They have a dog/cat question. It's the only reason they contact me."

My qualifiers for when you're being taken advantage of, and most rule-breakers fulfill two or three categories at once:

- They're not that good a friend.
- They ask multiple times for recommendations.
- They never speak to you socially otherwise.

- They're not even a client with your practice.
- They don't bother taking the advice you give.

If your friends/acquaintances fulfill any of those criteria, or a happy combination, welcome to veterinary medicine.

Living in this role just attracts the questioners. I would bet my pinky toe that everyone in the field has been the recipient of a shitty cell phone picture in their inbox of some nondescript blemish of uncertain anatomical location from their pal, querying for a free diagnosis. Or some similar variation.

If I'm feeling generous and like the questioner well enough, I may give them a little background into the possibilities of what that blurry blemish might be, but it always comes with the disclaimer that one doesn't diagnose from a photo. There's a list of rule-outs, and chances are fantastic I cannot definitively rule any of them out from your pixelated mess. I can't tell my pal across the country whether that spot is a lick granuloma or contagious ringworm, because I can't see it in person. Under good lighting. With hands-on interaction and palpation. In comparison with the rest of the animal, and its other vitals and symptoms. I don't have my diagnostic equipment to tell me what's happening on a cellular level. And, and, and. My ultimate answer is almost always:

"Take them to the vet."

Let's be honest. A few general questions on occasion are permissible. I like being helpful to allay concerns or manage expectations. But if buddy's asking for the full workup via phone? Resentment seeps in. If they're not making an appointment to actually take care of the problem, they're going to be labeled the cheap-ass in my book. And I'm less inclined to be helpful next time.

I and some of my cohorts in the field have comparable complaints about friends or casual acquaintances asking for free advice, while knowing full well that individual goes to our competing hospital down the street. In that instance? A brief inquiry is permissible. Then? They ought to take those questions to the staff who actually know Snowball. The ones they're paying for that veterinary-client-patient relationship. And to stop spitting in the faces of their friends by angling for services they know damn well should be paid for. Or at least buy them a nice bottle of wine for their time.

If they're asking after business hours? Hell, a little consideration goes a long way.

It's gotten to the point my husband has lost patience. We might be out at the pub, a restaurant, or other social affair, and someone comes to chat with me. "Hey, can I ask a vet question?" I'm not terribly popular otherwise, so it's almost expected that's the reason someone wants an audience with me. That said, I get tired of it, too. I've clocked out from the clinic and I'm ready to enjoy my Manhattan in peace. I'll strive for politeness and entertain the question for a few minutes. "No, I don't know anything about that supplement. It may not harm, but it may not help either … exactly, yeah, cause it's not FDA-regulated, and they can claim whatever they want on the label, so … hey, I love your necklace! Where'd you get that?"

Since they're not paying me for the consultation, it's time to change the subject. Trying to keep the marriage happy and whatnot. Husband just wants a night out with the wife, without having to hear about animal diarrhea.

I imagine this is not a unique problem to the veterinary world, but we get it bad. Other skilled professionals can surely relate. I've been messaged late and also *really late* sometimes. Most of them could have waited. I always appreciated more the people that prefaced their questions with, "Sorry to bother you about this so late, but ..." because at least they have awareness of it. When I trained new employees, I drilled into their heads to never give out their personal numbers to clients they didn't already know on a personal basis. It just never goes well. One of my top-spending clients always casually asked for numbers from whichever employee was scheduled to watch her boarding animals. The newbies were taught to dodge it with an offer of communication from our professional email instead. That particular client wanted to be able to text at will to ask how her cats were doing. She also had a history of pestering our manager in the middle of the night about appointments she wanted to make, because she was awake, thought of it, and didn't want to forget by morning. I'm entirely defensive about my personal time, and I guard that for those newer employees as well. We eventually had to tell that client—nicely—we don't give out personal numbers anymore. Once we finally said it, she was perfectly accepting. Might have even taken the hint to quit messaging the manager outside work hours. Even felt bad, apparently, since she's well made up for it since. Besides regularly expressing gratitude for our care of her pets, she often calls ahead of her arrival to take a coffee order for the staff.

I don't work after hours. I'm not on call. That's not to speak for every professional, but the rule is the same no matter what. Respect our personal lives. I'm an unapologetic believer that veterinary workers need to have time away from anything veterinary-related. We need it to recharge. To have other fulfillment.

Well, that was a tangent about respecting space. Not sorry. Gotta look out for my people. But let's get back to the money bit.

Free shit.

Some have the audacity to ask for it in person. Some of those same people are a bit unstable, to be fair. But it's still aggravating.

One such couple adopted an older dog and had its previous records—all done by the shelter—sent to us, to establish us as their vet. We went to the trouble of creating their account and filled the record with the applicable information. And then they just ... begged for free advice. We dreaded seeing their old beater car pull into the parking lot, while one spouse would chain smoke for several minutes and dump a pile of nasty cheap cigarettes in our parking lot. Then, they'd come inside with the dog, park themselves on the lobby bench, and negotiations would begin.

Could we just look at the dog? No, no, don't do a full exam! We don't have the money for the office fee, but could you just peek at her and tell us if you think her skin looks ok? I know you can't tell me that, but I'm just sayin' that you could just ...

For a brief window, we were patient. After that? Our staff determined quickly that we weren't going to do anything with this couple unless they paid for it upfront. They never gave a dime to our clinic. Just showed up intermittently over the course of several months. Hoping for advice on cheap products they got from a farm supply or somewhere else, that I'm not allowed to comment on. Patience wore thin. We quit answering their questions and instead repeated the broken record.

"We can't do anything for you without an exam."

Eventually they moved to a neighboring state. I only knew because I got a request for patient records by another vet clinic there. I made sure to put a note of explanation on that record before I sent it, that while I had limited information on shelter-performed preventive care for the poor dog, and the name of the owner, we had never actually done anything for the dog in an official capacity. I don't think the recipient was surprised, after having met the couple.

One client frequently delayed paying her bills by sending her kids in to pick up the terrier from grooming appointments. Kiddos weren't carrying the money, and mom knew we'd feel awkward demanding payment from pre-teens. She'd put off paying until the next time she wanted the dog groomed. Until we finally called her on it and set expectations of payment before service. Kid or no kid.

Another client in my big-city hospital paid for an exam on one of his dogs but had conveniently brought his newly-adopted dog along to the same appointment. Wasn't on the books. Just along for the ride. Moral support. But that soon turned into the less-than-sly request.

"Do you think Dr. Q could just *look* at my other dog, and ... no, not examine her, no! But just ... you know. *Look* at her. And if she thinks that she looks good, just give me a thumbs-up?"

I relayed the request, knowing damn well it was the by-the-book vet, and the answer would be a resounding, "Hell no!"

And it was. It was still fun to ask.

Idiot.

Boarding services are often fraught with logistical issues, and certainly, hard work. After all the effort it requires, one doesn't want to have to worry about compensation. I once had a woman call to schedule a stay for several pets, but whose story was filled with red flags. Details which didn't add up. Still, I took her information, noting her unasked-for insistence that payment wouldn't be a problem. She had a mama that could also help with the bill, she promised. If that didn't give me reason to investigate further, a little digging revealed her years-old, inactive file. Turned to collections for non-payment.

Cross-checks with another clinic in town regarding her pets' vaccine status, quickly resulted in another hint.

"She ain't gonna pay," the manager of the other clinic said, without preamble, nor any further prompting than the client's name. "And Mama ain't gonna pay you, either. She says Mama will. But Mama never pays."

Which meant I had the onerous, incredibly awkward task of trying to cancel the boarding reservation. Alas, the woman never answered my calls. With luck, she might have been a no-show. No luck for me, though. The day of her scheduled boarding, she finally contacted us again. Only to apologize for running late, but to say they'd soon be on their way. No mention of the missed calls.

Our owner veterinarian loves a good film quote. Usually Westerns, but plenty of other classics. Sometimes he and I quizzed each other over our favorite lines. That day of ill-fated boarding schedules was the day I gladly surrendered the phone call to him. He politely, but firmly, explained the situation to the woman; we had history of unpaid bills. Astounded at his forwardness, they promised they would pay *this* time.

Yes, but, what about the old bill?

The woman argued back, why would she bother to pay for a dog that died a long time ago?

At which point, the vet was delighted to utilize an obscure reference. The clients couldn't be bothered, so why should we? They didn't have the decency to pay the old debt. Therefore, he said, "… we never do business again. Not for shoelaces or a stick of gum."

There was shocked silence from the receiver when he hung up the phone.

By the way, if *The Shawshank Redemption* isn't in your top five films, you're wrong.

Boarding woes. Sometimes we actually get to the boarding part. In the late summer one year, we had a new client schedule to board his energetic young black Labrador for about a week while he had a temporary out-of-state job. The date of his return came, and he never showed to collect poor Jackal. No notification of a change in plans. We called multiple times, of course, to be met with silence. Jackal remained. Days passed with still no word from the owner, so what could we do but keep taking care of the dog?

The manager finally got ahold of him close to the two-week mark, by dialing out from our second line. We suspect he only answered because he didn't recognize it as our main number. He was out of town again, he informed her, and would be back for Jackal soon. And no, he couldn't pay a portion of the boarding fees over the phone, but he would take care of it when he got back.

In the meantime, though Jackal was a sweet dog by nature, he was sick of being cooped up. I didn't blame him. That dog ought to have been permitted to run miles each day, but such exercise just wasn't feasible for our facility. He started to become unmanageable on his walks. The stir-crazy Lab was so excited, he would throw himself onto me. I'm no weakling, but the enthusiasm was hard to contain. Hard to keep him down and avoid getting clawed up. Got to the point I would have to throw him off me, and I'm sure it looked super professional for any passersby to witness a vet tech body slamming a patient while trying to walk from parking lot to grass. (Slight exaggeration, but I could barely get him off me.) And once again, owner ditched our calls for days more. Now aware of both numbers.

By three weeks, I'd had enough. The dog had stayed fourteen *extra* days, and he was miserable. I was miserable. And furious. I called the owner's phone a final time, leaving a voicemail in a tone that surely dripped with venom, informing him if he didn't pick up Jackal by the end of the day, I'd be surrendering the dog to the shelter for abandonment.

Lo and behold, owner showed up that day. Miraculous! Day twenty-one. Didn't pay a dime of the boarding fees. He didn't have the money, which was why he'd not come back before. I wondered how long he'd have let it go, had I not called with my shelter threat. We were pissed about his dishonest intentions, of course, but glad to let Jackal go. The owner's account got turned to collections after three months of non-payment status.

To his credit, though, he was in the extremely small margin of folks who came back and settled everything, about a year later. He paid the collection agency what he owed them, followed by the hundreds he owed us. Every cent, and then for the exam he'd been currently requesting that year. That squared us away. I mean, we'd never board for him ever again. But if he pays up front for regular services, we're good.

Some clients will always have a harder time catching up. Financial problems, never ending. Or with budgets stricter than others. You never want to judge another's circumstances, but there are times when it still smacks you in the face.

Like the client who always struggled to afford their bills. When they arrived for the nail trim appointment, they'd casually mention it'd been weeks since they ran out of the dog's congestive heart failure meds, but hey—they borrowed money today just to afford the nails, so meds had to wait. Too expensive this time. After finishing at the front counter, they loudly browsed the lobby bulletin board for community advertisements of animals or other miscellaneous items, keeping a sharp eye out for "anything free?"

Most everyone deserves the loving comfort of a beloved pet, but it sucks when you know an already financially-strapped client is seeking to add to their burden. Especially when their existing creatures are going without essentials.

One gentleman showed up at my clinic late in the evening with what we knew was a sob-story, that he had come by before and been promised free flea prevention, through some sort of rebate or coupon deal. We hadn't seen the man in years, according to our extremely limited record, but he came across as somewhat volatile and more than a little unstable. Like a fight would break out if he didn't get something. We had no past notes about any such promise, but we made some about him after that. Explicitly stating any future product was to be paid for, as the clinic owner decided to give some complimentary samples to get him by. No loss on our part, and not worth a fight.

While that was more scary than laughable, there's still one other "free" request I find the most outlandish.

Maybe we can't give out free exams to your pet, but hey, what's the harm in trying to get a free exam for yourself? One medical professional is the same as the next, right?

I wish I was joking when I say we've had to remind clients we have no authority to give human medical advice, so could they please stop showing us their weird rash under their shirt?

Hoarding a Horde

> "Hoarding can never end, for the heart of man always covets for more, its raging appetites can only be quenched by the heavy sands of the grave."
> —Bangambiki Habyarimana, from *Book of Wisdom*

Every veterinary practice has a crazy cat client. Or two. Or five.

One of our cat ladies received a large family inheritance and, having no one else in her life to spend it on besides the obscene number of feral cats meandering on her property, decided she wanted to donate a portion of it to a good cause. That good cause ended up being our clinic, but more on that in a moment. I did the odd job of delivering prescription cat food to her house several times, so I can say I saw her hoard with my own eyes.

Home delivery is not an expected day-to-day task for a veterinary technician, by the way. In fact, we discourage personal errands to people's homes, because the requests tend to get deeper and weirder. It starts off as dropping off a prescription, but then becomes, "Can you grab the feral cat out from under my couch and vaccinate it?" However. When you live in a small town and that particular client cannot drive and donated a shit-ton of money to your clinic? Well, sometimes you draw the short straw and do the weird job. Damn exceptions.

She was a kind lady with a good heart, but all I will say is that whoever's turn it was to take her nine or twelve bags of cat food, always came back saying, "Oh my God, you wouldn't believe ..."

For her charity, though, our clinic was the recipient of several thousand dollars to what we called our "Good Samaritan Fund." Good Sam money was not something we advertised, but used at our discretion for needy and deserving clientele who couldn't afford necessary treatments. Allowable for dogs, but even better if used for cats, due to the donor's own personal interests. She never wanted credit. Preferred to be anonymous. Wouldn't let us share her name with the receiving clients, even for a thank you card. She also never asked to see proof of where her money went, but for good measure, we kept a record of every client ID number that used a portion of the funding, how much, and a brief description of the patient's need. No client was allowed to use Good Sam funds twice. We wouldn't have anyone taking advantage.

The feral cats probably ranged anywhere from ten to thirty running through her property at any given moment. No, her neighbors didn't appreciate it. To me, yes, it's too many. Far too many. Anyone that has reached those numbers almost certainly has a population of sick, viral-infested felines.

Another of our feline-fanatic clients likes to go on an annual vacation and drop off four to six of their favorites to board with us while they're gone. Trust me when I say they make half the building reek with their stench, and it's unsafe to put a cat from any other household in the same room. (As an aside, whenever they bring in a sick cat for us to examine, it's always their "favorite one." They probably have as many as the donor client.)

Unfortunately, compared to others we've seen, these still don't come close to the most shocking. Not many qualify as a "true" hoard, in the minds of veterinary or animal control personnel, who have seen the worst-case scenarios. Houses absolutely overrun. Litter, feces, and urine everywhere. Sometimes deceased animals, rotting in hidden corners or buried under piles of trash and animal waste. One man from my area was rumored to have died from complications caused by the ammonia-filled house amidst his already immune-compromising illness.

My supervising vet will tell you he's seen cat hoards of well over a hundred, so the one that I experienced didn't come close. That's perfectly fine by me. When it was my turn to experience a bad one? Upwards of sixty cats was still enough. And a couple of dogs, too.

I'm assuming a neighbor complained. Whether for the stench or the sheer number running around, I don't know. That detail doesn't matter much. Animal Control officers came, charges were pressed, and then there was the matter of dealing with it. At least for my sake, no one asked me to capture all the animals from the home. Photos of the heavily-publicized event were enough, through our local news outlets. The activist groups were thrilled to have their heroic moment, swooping in with their traps and sharing snaps of the process. I'll give them credit for the manually laborious task but pardon me if I'm still put off by their lack of tact. Peace-signs and grins in their proud social media posts. Meanwhile, in the background, someone was having the worst moment in their life documented for show.

I'm not making excuses for the hoarder. But I do call for understanding of what happened in this scenario, as it's probably similar to many other hoarding scenarios.

I didn't have to go to the house, but my clinic was called to help with the intake at our county shelter. I'd initially assumed it was just a casual check on a few cats. However, when we realized the magnitude, I had my assistants help me to prepare. This had to be organized. Our main objective was to assess. See what we were dealing with, and then the bombarded shelter director would formulate a plan based on our health recommendations. Charts custom-created, clipboards, cat gloves, cat net, extra scrub jackets, latex gloves, syringes galore, sedative, and euthanasia solution. With such a call, we expected most of the cats to be in terrible shape. Euthanasia would likely be the best course of action. Cheerful task, right?

I'm happy to do business with our shelter, but I had to bite my tongue with the activist volunteers that were present. Yeah, they did the hard work of the captures and going into the shitshow of a house. But the second we walked through the shelter door, their ringleaders were in our faces, asking what kind of treatments we planned for the cats. Touting their opinions. My biased feelings immediately made me grit my teeth. That wasn't what we'd come for. The activist groups weren't going to pay for any of the treatments they were suggesting we needed to perform for the hoarded felines. This was purely a mission to assess the situation and, if necessary, euthanize any too far gone and suffering. Treatment for the healthy-enough ones would be a later step. A step decided on between us and the shelter director.

If I sound like an insensitive ass about people who want to make a difference, you're welcome to think it. I can respect that people want to be the idealists who save everything. I was once, too. They can't, though, and I'll get to that later. But what I've learned is such groups often end up doing more harm than good. The one in question was a huge proponent for TNR programs. Trap-Neuter-Release.

I'm in the camp that firmly believes this is a waste of resources, money, and effort. More of a biologist's perspective. TNR cats run amok with other outdoor cats, killing absurd amounts of wildlife. Native birds suffer, especially. Feral behavior in perpetuity. Destruction of property and gardens. Not to mention the wealth of diseases these felines carry. Viruses and parasites. Some of which are transmissible to humans.

TNR serves more to make the volunteers feel like they're making a difference, than actually making a positive difference. The numbers of feral cats successfully sterilized don't come close to touching the apex of that mountainous problem, for starters. Someone smarter than me did the math, and even if every vet in the country tackled their fair share, we'd still fall drastically short. If you could somehow keep a closed community of feral cats in isolation somewhere, you might reduce just that population, but realistically? Those odds are not good. Then, consider the fact that the sterilized cats which *are* being released are likely becoming more docile, without their hormonal tomcat attitudes. They'll be more apt to tolerate other cats in their territory. Then come more cats.

See my dilemma, though? I'm in the awkward position of being part of the team that's often asked to help with a mission I don't believe in. Not only that I don't believe in it, but feel causes more harm than good.

Back to the shelter hoard.

The doctor, two alternating assistants, and I went in with the shelter staff. Thank fuck, the activist volunteers were shuffled elsewhere by then. One or two at a time, cat crates were brought to us in rotation. We pulled each one out to do a quick check. Assigned number, description, sex, approximate age, overall condition, and other recommendations.

Well, for starters, I soon found it was silly to bother with descriptions. They all had the exact same coloring. Every one. Of course they did. It was an incestuous hoard. What struck us next was the estimated ages. I expected we'd see a wider range, but that wasn't the case. They were young. Almost all of them. The majority, less than a year old.

Most shocking of all? They weren't in a godawful condition. Don't get me wrong. They stunk to holy hell. Some were covered in diarrhea or urine scald sores. They all had fleas. Tons were alopecic—missing hair—as a result of flea allergy dermatitis. But those were all relatively easy fixes. Nothing some good preventive care and TLC couldn't smooth over.

Only one was euthanized that day for health reasons. One, out of over sixty. A few had to be euthanized later, but over other circumstances.

Now, while most probably rejoice to hear the kitties were healthier than anticipated, it meant the already-full shelter was inundated. On one hand, the activists were delighted. On the other, one of the shelter board members who had come to take stock privately whispered to me her concerns about the practicality of the matter. Cost of funding for vet care, food, and space for the animals when cages were already full were all valid concerns.

"Are you *sure* only one needed to be put down …?" she vented.

Indeed, competing interests at play. When it comes to animal welfare, everyone's got an opinion.

In the end, the activist volunteers earmarked their favorites from the bunch. You know. The ones with quirky personality. Missing an eye, or most unique moustache marking. Something marketable for when it came time to adopt them out. They were quick to claim those, and then some, to lift some of the burden from the shelter. Since the story got so much attention in our small town, the shelter's plight was publicized. The community pulled together to make donations, both monetary and much-needed supplies. I made sure our clinic helped promote it. We also accepted donations toward the shelter's veterinary account with us. It's not sexy to talk about, but we had to be paid for our time and resources used. Time taken away from potential paying clients.

Our clinic received some fanfare for our assistance. We were sent thank you cards, along with donations to help pay the shelter bills. People in the community who knew us personally asked about it for weeks. A restaurant I frequented gave me a complimentary high-end cocktail the next time I was there, simply because they'd seen my picture shared in the action shot for the paper.

That sort of treatment almost made me feel guilty. I didn't feel as though we'd done much that was noteworthy, to be honest, other than countless consultative conversations with shelter staff about the care of those cats. We tried to help them spread their dollars as far as possible, without compromising care. It wasn't their fault they'd had this dumped on them.

So, back to the hoarders themselves. Was it their fault? Well, yeah. But damn my soft heart, I wasn't without sympathy in this case. It was just a situation that wasn't well thought out to start and then spiraled out of control.

The owner had initially gotten a few cats for company for a disabled family member. One cat may have already been pregnant when it was acquired. As for the two younger kittens? The owner didn't intend to breed them initially. They simply didn't have the money, right when they were of an age to be fixed. They had to postpone veterinary care in favor of other human essentials. Then, cats being induced ovulators the way they are—aka, fantastic and efficient breeding machines—did what cats do so well. Females can become pregnant as young as four months of age, though typically closer to six. Short gestation period of only sixty-three days. Then? Bam, accidental litter. Litters are, on average, 3-6 kittens, but it could be more, could be less. Those procedures were put off a little longer, because then their saved funds had to go towards more cat food and litterbox sand. Then, guess what? It happened again. And again. And before they knew it, they were overwhelmed trying to feed all the cats and kittens. Who could even think of spaying and neutering? And where would they start?

That's why all the cats were so young. That's how prolific of breeders they can be. Most of the problem population in the house was created in a relatively short window of time. It didn't take years and years to accumulate all the filth. Probably two years or less to have gotten themselves into that mess.

It's sad. The owner claimed they did ask for help from the low-cost spay and neuter organization in town to assist them. Probably asked family or other friends. I couldn't say. But I'm not surprised they weren't able to get enough help. No one prepares for a situation such as that.

It seems corny to end on this note, but there's nothing else to say, except keep your pets to a manageable number. Spay and neuter. Keep your pet cats indoors, at least primarily, for their safety and the good of your community.

For the Sake of Levity: Boo-Hiss

One of my clinics was located within the confines of a major pet goods store. That pet store, in addition to food and supplies for all things pet-related, was also known to sell pets themselves. Kittens, mostly. Some rodents. Birds. Other reptiles and exotics, too.

At this location, we had a jovial team in the veterinary hub. Most of us got along well with each other. And when you like your coworkers, you bond and joke with your coworkers. This was no exception. Sometimes joking turned into playing harmless pranks, like tampering with the *Employee of the Month* board, or googly eyes on inanimate objects.

My favorite "prank" was a simple one.

Wrapping up one day, I was conversing with a VA about the details of a case in the back treatment area, when the receptionist emerged from the front lobby, her face alight and flushed from laughing.

"What's so funny?" we asked.

She jerked her thumb in the direction behind her.

"Alright, that's hilarious, guys. Who put the rubber snake along the exam room door?"

We gawked at her. Then at each other, waiting for the other

to confess to the childish prank, but I didn't do it, and neither did the VA.

Our faces all turned from bafflement to recognition at the same moment.

"Oh, shit. Grab that snake!"

The reptile caretakers were relieved their escapee had been found safe.

For Shame

"Courtesy is as much a mark of a gentleman as courage."
—Theodore Roosevelt

I must briefly chastise my cohorts in the field. And it's about client education.

Let me remind you, I'm a complete introvert. I'm not scared of people, but I don't prefer most of them. As such, I'm certainly not the face of my clinic. Hiding in the lab or surgery room is much preferred. Meanwhile, our office manager is much more gregarious. Good at chitchat. A genuinely nice person. Funny. Fair, when it comes to matters of business. She's part of a charitable community group that does good deeds anonymously. I like to call them her secret Fight Club meetings. She even gifted me a car, as it had been a pay-it-forward item once given to her. In a small town, our clients know her by name and expect her to be the voice that greets them on the phone.

When I answer and identify myself, there's often an awkward pause before they say, "Wait, who is this?" Or the other frequent occurrence is they simply address me by her name instead, carrying on the conversation assuming I am her. I don't bother to correct them, unless it really is a personal matter requiring her attention. I'm content being behind the scenes.

With that said, I suck it up and talk to those clients when I need to. I have a professional phone voice, like anyone who has worked customer service long enough. Maybe it was the missing common sense from some of my big city client base that made me this way. Maybe it's because I'm married to someone in academia, but I am an adamant advocate for good client education, and it seems to be something sorely lacking.

There must be a trend of obliviousness among veterinary workers. I don't mean to insult anyone's intelligence, because I know those out there reading this have it in spades. The majority are undoubtedly far smarter than I am. But for a number, awareness is missing. I say that because they don't know how to communicate or aren't doing a good job of educating the clients they've earned. When I talk about awareness, I mean considering the individual (in this case, the client) they're trying to engage with, firstly. How does the vet professional act with them? Word choices, inflection, and body language? I mean, really understanding the headspace of the person across from them.

Sometimes it's listening. A good listener is worth their weight in gold, which is as cliché as fuck to say, but few people do it truly well. If you're one of those folks that can't wait for someone to pause from speaking so you can have a turn—you're a poor listener.

For the sake of fairness, I'll fill you in on a time when I crashed and burned on this. Early in my experience, there was a hectic day at work. Amidst the chaos, the receptionist placed one of the scheduled clients in an exam room at her appointed time. Receptionist neglected to update our software system to alert us to the client's presence, and with the exam room tucked away from the treatment zone's line of sight, the team assumed her to be a no-show. The normal expectation was to get a VA/VT in there within minutes, followed soon after by the vet. Alas, she waited for an hour, without even being acknowledged.

The receptionist apologized profusely when she realized her mistake. I was quickly rushed in next to try to make up for lost time, with a trainee in tow. It was late in the day; time to look forward to closing soon, after this hurdle of an appointment. I did a quick look-over of the tired woman's pet and inquired after any concerns to pass on to the doctor. She quickly said no, with telltale signs of eagerness to get on with things.

As was the expectation of that job, I reached for the brochure from our wall and began to launch into my business spiel about the benefits of the preventive care package our clinic could offer her.

Until she interrupted me.

"Please," she said, without any trace of malice in her voice. Just the resignation of exhaustion after she must have had a very long day herself. "Please, don't try to sell me something."

Well, say that to any introvert, and we're sure going to feel like crumpling deeply into a hole of ourselves to die. My cheeks probably flushed with embarrassment. Not only for the awkwardness, but because I was ashamed of myself. In that moment, she was imploring me to just be fucking real for a second. To be a human being, seeing another human. One that may have already had stresses to her day made far worse. Who knew what else she had going on? Didn't matter, really. We'd already started off on the wrong foot. To be forgotten in an exam room for an hour, before anyone noticed? And there I was, adding insult.

Job expectation be damned. The situation was plain in front of my face. She wanted the remainder of her appointment handled swiftly, and we owed her that much. To cut out the bullshit. I put the pamphlet away without any protest and agreed I'd let the doctor know she was ready. Back outside the exam room, I swallowed my humiliation to admit to my trainee I shouldn't have done that.

Sometimes listening is not only hearing what is being said but also reading between the lines of what is unsaid. Medical professionals have to consider the whole picture. Not that I've nailed listening perfectly in every case, but we must do better.

I'm ranting on this whole point because of the obscene number of times I've taken a few short minutes to give someone guidance, and the clients are astoundingly grateful. Usually, they're not even my regular clients. They're calling around because they need a specialist referral, or even another local veterinarian that handles X-type of patient cases. Some show up just to talk to a real human, needing advice. I don't mean to say I'm offering them something over the top, or worthy of charging a consultation fee. I very much believe in charging for the value of our time and expertise. I mean the very basics of a brief description of what they *might* expect from the appointment. Or giving them a name to look up. "You should call XYZ Hospital, and they're probably going to ask for ABC information. Tell them Rover needs LMNOP procedure, and they should be able to give you an estimate."

Cue the standing ovation.

Of those coming to my clinic for a second opinion, or a change in general, some of them told me their regular vet never took the time to explain things to them. The most basic of concepts, usually. *What are anal glands and why is my dog scooting? What the heck is this medication my other vet prescribed and why do I have to give it to my dog all the time? You mean my cat's condition is viral and a chronic thing?* Guys, I don't hold some genius coin. My friends in the field know those answers. Most clients don't, and there's no benefit to leaving them in the dark. Taking one to three minutes to explain what's happening with their dog's hind end, sometimes with the handy-dandy aid of anatomy resource books, has some of them looking at me like I'm the hero of the day. And it shouldn't.

Communication. If you're thinking, "Who has time for that in the appointment schedule?" then you're too overbooked. Sacrificing quality for quantity. In the long run, it's going to hurt end-of-day totals more than it helps. You'll have better compliance with your recommended treatments for having taken the time. Those clients won't go searching for another clinic out of frustration when they don't understand the diagnosis or treatment of their pet, or when they feel they're not being listened to.

In my first months of ever working in a practice, I had a drama-queen client tell me she wanted a clinic that would, "Treat me like a name, not a number!" I'd only met her thirty seconds prior, so I like to think the complaint wasn't directed specifically at me. Who knows. I've stepped on toes before.

In fairness, Drama Queen had a point, despite the childish fit she was throwing to make said point. And I've never forgotten it. No one wants to be Number Thirty-Seven of your day. Remembering names goes a long way to make a client feel respected and worthwhile. Much of the time I forget the human's name, but they'll more than forgive that if I greet their animal by name.

So, you've vowed to be better about saying names more. What else?

Sometimes the medical concept has been explained nicely enough, but for whatever reason, the implementation of your recommended treatment is unrealistic. Finances are one of the most common hindrances, but there are others. Like when the client is physically unable to get it done. We've probably all had that elderly client who couldn't treat their animal's ear infection. Or in one of my cases, the lady in her nineties with two broken wrists and a touch of senility. We had to wonder if we were doing the right thing in giving her the chance to treat her newly-diagnosed diabetic terrier. We were lucky if she remembered to give the insulin, and even more so if she did it properly. At one of her glucose recheck appointments, she cheerfully told us she'd struggled with the subcutaneous injection, but —not to worry! She'd simply applied the insulin topically, instead. Figured doggo would get some good absorption that route.

Yes, sometimes difficult conversations are in order. But hey, use their name and it'll be so much more palatable!

Working in a small town, I know a number (ha!) of my clients personally, outside of the job. Sometimes that makes it more awkward to see their animals and their sense of ownership. Sometimes it's a privilege to witness. One such couple in the latter category was told their dog had developed a condition needing specialist attention. More than we could offer. All we could do was keep Scout comfortable and essentially, put a Band-Aid on the problem. I gave them all the information I could about the recommended referral. When I personally checked in with those friends/clients a few days later, they confided they'd looked into it but couldn't afford the specialist visits. It was obvious they felt remorse in telling me. I reassured them with a few short messages they weren't bad people by any means, despite their anxiety. That we would manage the condition medically and keep their sweet Scout comfortable. Later that week, a bottle of my favorite scotch showed up at the clinic, for me. (Not to brag, but I have good taste. Not a cheap bottle.) Just because I took a few moments to be real, as a human being. To ease their guilt. It meant more to them than I had realized.

We don't expect gifts or tips from our clients, ever. But I won't lie when I say it means a lot to us to receive thank you cards or other sentiments of gratitude. Lunch, baked goods, homemade jam, cheese plates, alcohol, flowers, massaging foot rollers, the best avocados in town, and even artwork have been gifted to the team for caring about pets. It's our job, but client appreciation goes a long way to balance out the stress. And gives us the warm fuzzies.

We give back when we can. A single-episode client showed up once, after a traumatic family event. She had a sibling who had just been incarcerated and wouldn't be coming home for the foreseeable future. During the sibling's imprisonment, their children and pets needed to be looked after. It fell to this poor woman.

With the events still fresh, it was apparent she was barely holding in the emotional stress of having nieces and nephews and dogs dumped on her. She was taking on the familial obligation as best she could. Just a sad situation. We did the necessary exam on the dogs, but what I recall most about that appointment was that it was approaching closing time when we finished.

Fuck it, we decided. Once off the clock, the doctor made an offer of a toast of acknowledgment, and the client gratefully accepted. All of us teary-eyed, we poured a round of whiskeys. For the sake of camaraderie. For the sake of humanity. To listen to a stranger and sympathize with her plight. Never saw her again, but that didn't matter. I hope she felt listened to that night.

Inside the Joke

"I love inside jokes. Love to be a part of one someday."
—Michael Scott from *The Office*, Season 3, Episode 2

There must be a word for that inside joke that originated from hearing something shitty someone said, and it's still inappropriately funny to repeat again and again. If someone can tell me what that word is, I'd be thrilled.

Mine doesn't even involve swearing, believe it or not.

It was the lead veterinarian for the whole region of hospitals. I couldn't even tell you what his title was. He was my boss's boss, and I never liked the guy. He was the one that came in and made sure to always find something wrong so he could call you out on it. I never heard him say anything nice. Some call it constructive criticism, sure. In his case, I called it being a condescending prick. He wasn't there except for once in a great while, so in my mind, he had no right to take on the role of mentor to any of us.

Yeah, I know that's how the hierarchical chain-of-command works. I can still think the guy's a prick.

Anyways. At one of those hospitals that has preventive care packages, of course Boss Vet's own dog was enrolled in the highest category. The package plan included the works. Full vaccines, dewormers, heartworm test, fecal exam, tonometry, senior bloodwork panel, and the standard three views of screening thoracic radiographs. We'll call doggo Chuckles, this time. Boss Vet chose my hospital's location to drop Chuckles off when routine updates were due. He let us know when he'd be back to pick him up, post-meetings. No other special requests. No concerns mentioned for Chuckles. Just asked us to complete the standard items.

We did everything on the list, squeezed into our typical busy day.

A quick note about my regular supervising doctor that day. Let's just say Dr. Z. He was the most level-headed, patient man I've ever worked with. If you had a stressful scenario, or a difficult client who needed to be talked off the ledge, Dr. Z was the veterinarian you wanted. A calming presence.

Boss Vet eventually came back to pick up Chuckles but of course took the liberty of perusing the records himself. He could walk around like he owned the place. Checked the notes, the bloodwork results, and then went to view the radiographs on our digital monitor. The X-ray machine was located around the corner from the main treatment area, where I was presently working on another patient with Dr. Z.

Boss Vet called over to Dr. Z, inquiring as to whether we'd seen any red flags on Chuckles. Z answered no. A few seconds passed in silence while Boss Vet clicked through the three radiograph images of Chuckles' thorax. We assumed he was content, until he voiced his next concern.

"What, are there no hips rads?" Boss Vet called again, from around the corner.

Dr. Z's brow furrowed in confusion. Taken aback.

"I … no? We did the three chest films …"

"Well, he's a golden retriever, Z! Some hips rads would've been nice."

In response to that most passive-aggressive complaint, for the first and only time I can remember, Dr. Z had a brief lapse in professionalism. His quiet expression turned to what can only be described as profound disgust toward the senior vet, as he mouthed the words to me.

What the fuck?

What else was there to say? I had to bite my lip to not bust up laughing. Grateful Dr. Z was human enough to allow himself to be annoyed. Annoyed at the audacity that man possessed, to complain about us not reading his mind and adding more to the procedural list for Chuckles. Items that would have cost any other client extra. How presumptuous would we have had to be?

Any time after, if we wanted to make each other laugh, Dr. Z and I would shoot that line at each other with as much condescending disdain as we could muster.

"What, you didn't bring me a coffee this morning? Pfft. *Would've been nice.*"

Or,

"Dr. Z, what's this? I noticed you didn't wrap any of these surgery packs that are normally my job to do. Pssht. *Would've been nice.*"

Of course I told the story to my spouse, and it's been well-incorporated into our regular wheel of inside jokes. Years later, we still say it for any absurd request. Would've been nice if people didn't suck.

Stay Classy

"Our weakness as humans, turns out to be, in a way,
our strength. We are totally gregarious, social animals,
we absolutely need each other …"
—Dr. Biruté Galdikas

My manager prides herself on running the best-smelling veterinary clinic in our town. Cleanliness and organization are among her top priorities. She keeps an impressive collection of air fresheners, scented plug-ins, and essential oils for diffusers. Utilized in good balance, of course. Not all running at once.

Where animals are, bad odors happen. Multiple times a day. Yeasty skin conditions, ear infections, bodily fluids, excretions, vomitus, necrotic masses, dental disease that could knock a horse over … many possibilities. I've got a strong stomach, normally. Hell, I can eat my lunch anywhere in the clinic. But as the tech, I'm often the one coming face-to-face with the source. If you scrolled my colleagues' photo rolls, you'd find some unflattering snaps of me with cotton balls shoved in my nose during the most undesirable circumstances.

All-time worst was the weekend shift I worked solo, when an elderly client delivered his deceased dog for cremation.

From the back of a truck bed, I hauled in the heavy, loosely tarp-draped body that had been baking in the sun for more than a day. Had the pleasure of trying to bag the creature, ungainly huge and with leaking bodily fluids dripping everywhere. The stench of decay filled the office. Meanwhile, I was within an inch of puking. Simultaneously, still running back and forth to answer reception phone calls. Like a bad sitcom episode. Shame there was no laugh-track.

I digress. Our staff work hard to eliminate odors efficiently.

Manager is always pleased when a new visitor walks in the door and exclaims at how pleasant the building smells, compared to the olfactorily-offensive experiences they've had at the other clinics. I've heard the comment several times.

"Oh, it actually smells *good* in here!"

With any luck, they halt their observations there. In other cases, they go on to tell us exactly which other vet hospital literally stank. Or, figuratively. There's many an uncomfortable time a new client expounds further on a negative experience from elsewhere. Bashing a doctor, a distrusted diagnosis, a protocol they didn't care for, feeling like a number, scheduling booked out too far, or any number of scenarios. For whatever reason, we hear disparaging comments about our veterinary neighbors.

At that point, it's easy pickings to chime in with agreement. To repeat something condescending, or to turn it around and boast why we do it better.

Here's my SOAPBOX moment to say, veterinary professionals should *never* be bashing other professionals. Not to the clients. It's the very definition of marking yourself as the unprofessional one.

I'm not saying I don't have opinions about some. I do. Prior to my employment at my current facility, I'd been a client with two other hospitals for my personal pets. I could rant about what terrible communicators they were for surgical appointments, or how dismissive a certain veterinarian was to deal with. But I don't. Not to the client in front of me. It's a basic professional courtesy, and it ought to be the standard between facilities. I mean, high school was miserable enough, do we need to keep up the gossip-mongering cliques as adults?

Yes, we're a business, and you might argue we're in competition with the other places. To an extent, sure, I guess. But it happens far more frequently that we rely on each other, so why would I jeopardize the working relationship? Sometimes our doctor has to be out of town, so I might ask the favor that they see one of my regulars urgently. They might have had an influx of suspected parvo cases that week, and the receptionist calls us to ask if they could borrow two of our parvo tests. It just makes sense to be on good terms with each other. It's not often we'd be in a situation of having a client shortage. There's plenty of business to spread between us.

When clients bad-mouth another place, my typical strategy is to avoid engagement with that aspect of the discussion. I deflect and turn it back to the concern they have for their pet, only responding with our own recommendation, without the side-by-side comparison. Ignoring the bashing comment, I just focus on the case symptom.

"Oh, so if you're noticing Garfield is peeing outside the box, we suggest …"

The only time I may point out those comparison details, is if our clinic's protocol is the same as the other's. That's the exception I have for drawing attention to it. A solidarity move.

"I'm sorry you had a bad experience over there, but we would actually have the same scenario with our boarding schedule, and the reason is …"

Hey, like we discussed a few chapters ago? Sometimes it just comes back to communication. How you deliver your bad news, or whether you tell them anything at all. I earned a client once, who had been told by the "other" clinic her dog would never be allowed to board again, due to its high anxiety and destructive behavior. Why did I win her over? Just because I took time to explain what problems arise with challenging boarders. What unsafe scenario might have happened for the other place to come to that conclusion. Hell, I even told her straight, my clinic would not be able to board her dog, either. I trusted the file notes they'd sent me. Flags and alerts all over it. We would have the same issues, almost certainly, I told her, because we follow nearly the exact pattern of boarding care. Yet because I took the time to speak with her respectfully about the process and expectations, she switched her services to us. No, we don't board for her, but we deal with all other aspects.

She felt listened to. That was the only real difference in her care between our facility and the one across town.

Fact is, though, we love it when there's camaraderie between vet facilities. When I see the name of The Other Clinic come up on our caller ID, sometimes I hold my breath for a second of hopefulness. Then answer with our clinic greeting and my name.

"Oh, thank God it's you," the long-time receptionist from the Other Clinic always gushes. The voice I'd hoped for, in return. She says that to me and the manager only, when we're the ones taking her call. And she means it. Because we're straight with each other. She'll rant about her shit-show of a day if she's got time. (Her day is always a shit-show. She'll make time to tell us about it.) Trusting us with details about her vets who aren't getting along, staffing frustrations, or the latest disaster client. Sometimes that is the most valuable courtesy we extend, between the clinics. If someone was an especially heinously behaved client or tried to scam their way out of paying the bill, we'll give our neighbors a heads up. They return the favor.

"Add Jane Doe to your watch-list. She still owes us, and she's gonna be calling you next. You'll never see a dime from her. She'll lay on the guilt trip, too."

It isn't always outright anger we hear. Sometimes when a potential client wants to give our clinic a try, or to get a second opinion, they feel incredibly awkward about it. I think it's human nature to *not* want to express displeasure to another. The nature of *kind* people, at least. It's uncomfortable to say you weren't satisfied with the service. Or, as in my small town, I'm certain each veterinary location has their fair share of clients who come to them out of a sense of obligation. They know the vet or someone on staff personally, so they feel they ought to be patrons. A double-edged sword, more often than not. Alas, we get the occasional episode of someone feeling guilty about going to "the competitor." Maybe even trying to be covert about it. I've asked new clients to bring previous records with them, or request they be sent to my clinic, and have been met with resistance. They're too embarrassed to ask the primary clinic—do I *really* have to have the record?

Depending on the clinic of origin, sometimes I can ask for them, sometimes not. Some will have policies that only owners can make the request.

As one lacking in social confidence, I'm not without sympathy to this plight. The squirmy feeling of your go-to finding out you're flirting with someone else? The injustice of it all!

No, really. If it's any consolation to the nervous client, especially among hospitals in the same town or city, we clinics transfer records back and forth constantly. Numerous times a week. A day. We seldom take it personally. It is a business, your animals have needs, you have a busy schedule, and so do we. Sometimes you want another pair of eyes on the problem. See if the professionals are in agreement. We get it. A good number of my regulars have regular accounts at my neighbors' places, too. Often comes down to which pet needs care. Or who has more convenient availability when they want it. So long as we're not recommending contradicting therapies, or there's a situation that calls for great consistency in care, it's usually fine.

To my neighboring vet friends, even if our surgical protocols or flea-prevention recommendations sometimes differ, I do care about you. I choose to see you as a business ally, rather than an enemy. We joined the same profession, for the same mission of animal health and welfare. How idiotic would it be to view each other with disdain? When the client complains about you, I'll stand in your corner. I wasn't there for the appointment to see how your patient presented. I didn't hear what was recommended, nor how the client responded to it. When I hear that complaint, I'm extending to you the professional courtesy of assuming you have a side of the story, too. That your decision on that day, at that time, with the knowledge you had, was based in sound logic. Even if our clinic's assessment or recommendation contrasts, negative reviews of you will not be voiced by me.

I hope you'll do the same for me and my team, when the occasion is presented to you. It will. It already has.

Even more than the teams of outsiders, it's critical to be a team player on your home turf. I want to trust the person restraining the animal —that I'm about to poke with a needle—knows what they're doing so I don't get bitten in the face. If your restraint is lacking, I'll let you know. Promise. And in every other aspect, I want to trust those fellow staff to do their jobs well.

Our hope is to have clients and pets satisfied with the services and care received. To know our people can deliver that to said client. That's a given. But at the end of the day, *my* people come first. So, when a team member's integrity is called into question by an upset client, often you need to be ready to defend your person. It's the classy move—additional brownie points for delivering the message with honesty and professionalism. Bluntness, as needed.

We once received a complaint from a regular client about a scheduling response given by one of our VAs. There were clearly hopes of us "correcting" the perceived issue. Basically, they weren't offered the weekend appointment time they wanted, or felt they were entitled to. Decided our VA had been rude to deny them. They expected we'd put her in her place, or perhaps an even more drastic disciplinary measure.

Other staff were initially sweating the issue, when we heard the clients had been pissed off. I suppose I have far less patience. Scoffing at the idea of licking their shoes.

"I'm not throwing [VA] under the bus for doing exactly what she was told to do," was my stubborn response.

That was the end of the discussion. The VA had been given specific instructions by her superiors on our limited weekend

scheduling and had followed that guidance. What more was there to say? She's also a very soft-spoken, thorough, and polite person, and I wasn't going to even entertain the notion she'd been rude to them. Clients just didn't like the answer, even delivered by a kind individual. They could fuck off. Or come back when they calmed down.

The most egregious case was a client who once practically campaigned against a receptionist I worked with. The receptionist was regarded by our team as a good, kind person, and an absolute genius at the administrative workings of the job. We were fortunate to have her. The client was a man who was both particular by nature, and also deeply passionate about his dog. That's the kindest description I could lend him.

To all other intents and purposes, he was an ass.

Oh, don't get me wrong. The dog was lovely. We liked the dog. Polly Princess Puffington may have suffered an absurdly ridiculous name, but she was an adorably sweet wire-haired terrier-mix. And no, that wasn't her actual name. You should know by now I use aliases here, but the real dog's name was very much in the same vein. She wasn't bequeathed it by a six-year-old, either. Our adult client chose that all on his own.

I didn't get to witness the fateful incident, but I heard about it, as did everyone else—what a wretched person our receptionist was. Polly Princess Puffington had a drop-off appointment one morning, and during the hand-over of said pooch from owner to our dear receptionist, the client was displeased. *Manhandled*, he insisted. His darling dog was carelessly, recklessly grabbed—manhandled!—by our receptionist when she took Polly from him. And thus, the personal vendetta began.

The client overall liked our facility. Liked the veterinarians. Even liked the other receptionists pretty well. Except for that notable one, whom he learned by name. The Manhandler. And for that reason, he made bullying demands and manipulative requests surrounding his appointments for Polly Princess Puffington that we put up with for, frankly, too long. Calling to dictate he was coming for such-and-such appointment, but, "Ma'am," he would say. "That girl, [receptionist]? She's not to touch my Polly. That girl manhandled my dog, ma'am, so I want to make sure [other receptionist] is the one that takes her back. Can you make sure of that?"

We'd try to smooth it over. To assure him she was a good person who treated pets well, but he couldn't be persuaded. Finally, the Chief of Staff had had enough and set the terms.

Manhandler did not manhandle Polly, he told the client. (No, he didn't call her "Manhandler." Just imagine the receptionist's name. Keep up.) Manhandler was a valued member of our team, and we weren't going to tolerate his abusive personal attacks any further. If he wished to continue bringing Polly Princess Puffington to be treated as our patient, he was going to have to civilly accept Manhandler in her role. Take it or leave it.

That client didn't want to leave, as it was hard for him to find vets he liked and trusted. He told us as much. Still, he struggled to meet those 'cruel' terms. What to do? Aha! He ceased his damning vocal rants against our poor receptionist, yes, but came up with an alternative tactic for a while. Physically arriving at the location and (unsuccessfully) hiding out, with Polly under his arm, to see who was working the front desk. If it was Manhandler? Nope. Slink out the side and try another day. If it was Other Receptionist? Green light! He could just so happen to be in the neighborhood, and wondering if we might be able to work Polly into our schedule that very day? And, oh! Manhandler wasn't there? Darn the luck. Well, how was he to know? He was cooperating, though! No rules broken. He'd prove how friendly they were another day, perhaps.

... Yeah, the Chief of Staff wasn't too impressed, either. He urged the client again to shape up, or the already-thin ice would finish cracking all the way.

Most begrudgingly, the client managed to give in and give our receptionist another chance with Polly. His love for the veterinarian just barely won out. But soon after, he was moving halfway across the country, anyway. I heard about the anxious call to our clinic where, as luck would have it, his least-favorite receptionist answered the phone. It was almost as if he'd called for a truce, relaying to her his fears of finding a good vet in his new state. Wondering if we might somehow know who to suggest in that area.

"I think we both know you're particular on what you like, don't we?" she answered him. "Even if we knew them, you'd want to make up your own mind."

"Yeah, I know," he said in near-defeat.

We had no idea about any vets that far away, but in an act of extraordinary kindness, the former enemies had a lengthier conversation about what approach he might take to find a good veterinary service for Polly when he got settled.

That case sort of worked out in the end, but it took a little longer than I would have liked. We should have put our foot down and stood up for our team member sooner.

And if it comes down to it, stand up for yourself, if the occasion calls for it.

Some clients have white-coat syndrome. They're nervous about chatting with the veterinarians, but they'll open up to the techs. Others are the opposite, seeing techs as a speed bump and wanting to go straight to "the source." Goes both ways. One time, a knowledgeable client who was a regular dog rescuer arrived for her appointment and was subtly unexcited not to see her regular vet. The relief vet was a lovely person, but petite in build and unimpressive as an authority. I'd already gathered an initial history, in which the client assured me she had no specific questions. When the vet and I both returned to the room, client began a tirade of obscure medical scenario grilling. After having said the client had no concerns, I was mortified, angry at the lie and disrespectful "testing" of the young vet, who thankfully was cool and composed.

When we left the room, I apologized to her profusely. Swearing that none of those questions had been mentioned. I wasn't meaning to be a saboteur. Vet wasn't upset at me, thankfully. Sadly, she was somewhat used to her credibility being questioned, due to her stature.

One of my clients is an absolute control freak and tries to micromanage everything. Condescension thick in the air with every interaction. Another case of Love-your-dog-but-can't-stand-you. If Mr. Congeniality has a medical concern about doggo, he second-guesses anything you recommend or wants to know why you can't give him a more in-depth answer. To a neurotic degree. Why can I suggest his dog has an overgrowth of cocci bacteria from my ear swab cytology, yet I can't tell him the precise species of cocci? Well, why don't we have the equipment to tell him that?! How can we know the antibiotic is correct?

My favorite moment with Mr. Congeniality occurred when he happened to enter the lobby at the same time as a genuinely nice-guy client. Nice-Guy politely allowed our less-than-charismatic friend to go before him, and then got to witness the exchange we had. The one in which Mr. Congeniality tried to dictate exactly how I'd be walking his dog while it was boarding, as I surely didn't know his dog was special, and needed to be walked with X-length leash so doggo could sniff and explore to his heart's content! How was I going to hold the leash on my arm? And here's what kind of attachment it should have to the collar. And how many times a day was this going to happen? For what length of time? And, and, and.

Though not thrilled with my own pushy insistence I was qualified to walk a dog, he eventually surrendered his pet and left. I hadn't made any loud statements, but neither was I going to cower and answer to his bullying. I held my ground on what I would do, in compliance with our boarding policy.

"Wow. Maybe he shouldn't be taking his dog out in public, if it's so special," remarked Nice-Guy, after the troublesome one left.

I wanted to high-five him in agreement but settled for plastering on my customer service smile. Thanked him for his considerable patience and asked how I could help him.

The majority of clients are friendly enough. Worthy of gold stars in behavior school. Alas, we've had more than a few who ought to have been asked to consider taking their services elsewhere. Bottom line? No one ought to be bullied in this career. Nor to be the bully. If you've got a personnel issue, or more training is warranted, deal with that swiftly. But in the meantime, protect yourself. Look out for your fellow staff. And honor the folks on the other side of town fighting the same battles as you.

If you've been that vector of negativity before, change it. Simple as that. Have your vet friends' backs. I'm not asking.

For the Sake of Levity: To-may-to, To-mah-to

I'm not the most brilliant at anything, but anatomy is just fun for me. Hard for me to fathom that it's not as exciting for the next person. Even more so, it's a marvel when fully-fledged adults miss basic concepts.

One day I'm collecting my patient history in the exam room with my two clients. They're a young-ish couple. Late twenties, early thirties. The wife is doing all the talking about the beagle sprawled out on the floor, and I'm taking the relevant notes, while also doing my best to keep her on task. Husband? He's clearly bored out of his mind. Slouching posture like a sullen teenager who's been dragged along to the appointment.

Wife is a talker. Rambling on and on, while husband is staring off into space. At a certain point, she remembered to ask us to trim Clifford's nails. Which led to her long-winded complaint about her mother, who fails to get it done frequently enough for her own pooch.

"... And my mother! Lord, she just needs to do it more often! I know that's so painful for the dogs, and her poor dog's nails are so overgrown. I would do it for her, but I'm scared to do it. I know there's that part of the nail you're not supposed to cut into, and ... oh, what's it called ...?"

I opened my mouth to answer her query, but didn't get the chance for my volley in the conversation. She did it herself first, with assured confidence.

"Oh, right! The clit."

With my mouth already open to speak, my jaw probably didn't have much further to drop. In contrast, the husband's glazed-over eyes suddenly became more alert. Widening in horror. His head turned on his neck like a swivel as he gawked at his wife. As astounded as me.

One of us had to be the hero, so I tried to move past my surely-beet-red face.

"Oh ... oh, that's ... so close. *Quick* is the word you're thinking of. You don't want to cut into the dog's quick ..."

I'm sure he explained it to her as soon as I left the room, and I'm just as sure she was mortified. Meanwhile, I was childishly galloping to go tell one of my coworkers and so upset that they were all too busy to listen. To this day, it's my favorite misuse of anatomical terms.

Bearing False Whiskers

"You can speak with spiritual eloquence, pray in public, and maintain a holy appearance … but it is your behavior that will reveal your true character."
—Dr. Steve Maraboli

I grew up in a religious household, despite any appearances to the contrary.

Whether or not I've remained the most pious in the faith of my childhood is irrelevant to this venture. What is relevant to establish is that I'm content to coexist with my fellow humans, regardless of what they believe in. So long as no one's harmed, of course. Important caveat.

Religion shouldn't be something intruding much in my place of work. But since I'm writing this, you know it has come up.

My boss is a God-fearing person. That shouldn't be relevant either, but in a small town, plenty of folks know him by reputation or from their mutual church activities. What quickly became apparent when I started working for him was the propensity of people to try to use his devout faith against him in business. Or rather, to take advantage. Thus, while I want to respect anyone's right to believe—or not—in the theology of their choosing, it's nothing short of aggravating to witness religion used as a tool of manipulation.

Preying on the good nature of others is the scam that comes into play. No "praying" pun intended.

Why does another's creed come into play in my office? Ties back into another all-too-common issue. I answer multiple phone calls a day where people begin with, "Let me tell you my situation." And you hope whatever comes next in the conversation is something fixable. We all like to be the hero with the solution. Duh. What's never an easy fix is when the client or potential-client says they have no money, or don't get paid until the end of the month, so could they just charge until …?

The sob story is often the build-up to an emotional guilt-trip.

We have a policy against charging, precisely because too many people never paid what they promised. Ruined it for the rest. We make quiet exceptions if and only if they've been a long-standing client and proven their good faith.

A lot of folks don't like to admit they have financial constraints. It's a touchy subject. We hate to talk about it, too. Anytime payment is fraught with issues. None of us in the veterinary field got into it because we like to talk about money, but unfortunately there's a business aspect we can't ignore. It's happened too many times that we finish the entire appointment and have all the medications ready to go before the client finally tells us at check-out they have no money. Then, it's doctor-discretion as to how we handle it. Do we feel sorry enough for the pet that desperately needs the prescription, so we forgo the fees for our services so they can skate by? Or are we going to be hardasses about it, and demand the service be paid for, before sending home any goods?

If we accepted every request for an IOU, we'd have to close our doors. Straight up. We have bills to pay, too. Products, staff salaries, insurance, licensing fees, equipment maintenance, and so on. None of those items can be charged indefinitely. Not to mention the challenge of staying competitive in our surrounding market and competing against outside pharmacies and pet suppliers.

We want to save everything that comes through our doors, but without consistent payment, that's not a reality.

What does finance have to do with religion? Let's get back to the fishing phone calls for a second. For some who didn't like to admit their budgeting woes upfront, we heard a frequent claim, tied into personal beliefs.

"I heard that Dr. A is a Christian? They say he's someone that actually *cares* about animals? We're *Christians*, ma'am. And see, I've got this dog ..."

I feel my neck get hot. Maybe my eye starts twitching. Not because I inherently take issue with faith. On the contrary. But they've just convicted themselves. I wish it wasn't the case, as that's an embarrassing abuse on behalf of all the actual good Christians. These callers give a bad name to the faithful flock. Because when someone called and specifically referenced Dr. A's Christian position, I learned it was code for two things:

1. They have no money.
2. They want free shit.

I have no other way to sugarcoat that. The front desk picked up on it quickly and would have to try to sidestep drama. Those calling with this script, or variations of it, played up the religious angle in hopes of winning emotional points. In an effort to manipulate us into giving away business, with the subtle threat of tarnishing our Godly-status if we didn't cooperate with their requests. After all, did we want to be lumped in the category of un-Christian Dr. X's clinic down the street, who must surely hate animals? That must be the logical explanation for heathen businesses refusing service, without money upfront.

Me? I call that accuser a wolf in sheep's clothing. Really rather un-Christian.

No matter which God you pray to, it's insulting to those of us who dedicated our lives and daily endeavors to the betterment of animal health. In case you needed a reminder, I'm talking about people like the wonderful vet I watched break down into tears of guilt, after learning from a specialist that she had misdiagnosed her feline patient's X-ray results. Questioning her worth and credentials because of a mistake that affected the patient's treatment. Trying to swallow emotion and regroup for the next patient. Or, my formidable fellow RVT, whom I once witnessed remove her own scrub top, tearing it into strips in order to stabilize the degloved leg of a shepherd that had charged headlong into a tree stump. Effectively tearing the skin away from muscle, like a sock bunched loosely around an ankle. (RVT had a tank on underneath, don't make it weird.)

That dog wouldn't even be her patient; she was just sending him on to the next facility because ours wasn't equipped to handle the emergency. The literal shirt off her back. We fucking care.

I don't have a miraculous solution for people in a tight financial spot. I just ask for understanding when we say we can't allow for charging, we really can't. We wish we could. We wish we could treat everything with the best care. That it was free or at least affordable for everyone. We hate to see something go untreated when we know we could have helped.

That said, it'll go a long way for folks to be upfront and honest with us. We've heard all the manipulation tactics and sob stories. I'm much more appreciative and inclined to try to help figure something out if they come in right away and say, "Hey, I've only got twenty bucks to spend," rather than trying to guilt me for twenty minutes before getting to that crucial point. Can't make promises, but maybe I've got a coupon for that prescription food to help get to next payday. Maybe I can find a cheaper deworming alternative than the gold standard. Just maybe I had a donation of personal effects brought in when another client's pet passed away. Or, maybe a suggestion (what the pharmacy companies don't want us to tell you) of sizing up in the weight category of monthly prevention doses, by splitting a big dose in half and sharing it between two smaller pets for more mileage. That's cheaper than buying individuals for each pet.

—

Quick tangent, on that pharmaceutical issue of splitting the dose. The reasoning I hear from drug reps is they can't guarantee even distribution of the active ingredient, throughout the whole pill. Maybe. Makes for a sound argument. But when there's a financially-strapped client in front of me begging for a solution, it seems like a better calculated risk than the pet going without entirely, or the client buying some cheap shit from Wally-World that doesn't work. That's a more tragic waste of precious funds.

Drug companies offer rebate incentives for buying products in bulk package deals, with the caveat that the listed patient's weight has to match the product size. So, if I try to sell Product XYZ meant for dogs weighing between 50-100 pounds, but they see Squeakers only weighs 37 pounds on my patient chart, the rebate is gonna get rejected. I'm not a fan of this policing. In any case, my client asking if they can just buy one pill and split it in half can't come close to affording the whole package-deal rebate, so I might as well help them get by. Also? The pharmaceutical companies get cheaper and more exclusive about those rebate offers with every passing year. I said what I said.

—

Back to the point. Clients? Work with me. I'll try to work with you, and if I can, make it happen. Don't invoke a deity into the conversation.

We had one regular client—and I do mean *had*—that abused the faith-based arguments for their veterinary services, to an insane degree. One of the most shamefully behaved people I have encountered. And let me state this individual was a Church leader. As in, the head of his congregation. Giving spiritual guidance.

Frankly, this man was just a bad veterinary client. I can only hope he was a better minister to the notion of divine salvation.

The Preacher was not a comfortable person to be around. Some folks have that gift of the warm, welcoming vibe, or the ability to chat freely and easily with anyone. I'm not one of them, either, but I hope I at least don't make your skin crawl when we occupy the same room. Nothing the Preacher ever said in my general direction felt sincere.

His jokes never landed. He would try to banter, but it felt as though he might have memorized conversational lines to use with other humans. And he usually repeated the same one. A miserable attempt at being charming, I'm sure. At the end of every appointment, at the lobby desk, we were treated to the routine:

"Every time I deal with a woman, it costs me money!"

There might have been polite chuckles by some of my nicer coworkers to start, but that would be generous. Eventually, I don't think any of us could muster up the customer service laugh. If he was lucky, he might have gotten a nostril flare and expulsion of air. Uttering anything else would have been more than I could bear for that man.

Only one staff member in our clinic is a man—the older doctor who owns the practice. The veterinary field is becoming a more female-dominated place, no matter what role. Men as coworkers are rare these days. Why? Several factors, but some of the commonly understood reasons are that the profession calls for nurturing personalities, which is a trait more attributed to females. While women have been allowed in the field for some time, setting the example for future generations, the increase in our numbers didn't come until the 1970s, thanks to elimination of discriminatory admissions in schools. Somewhere soon after 2000, the number of women surpassed men. Currently, private practices are increasingly being bought out by corporations, which tends to be a drawback for males. More often, men seek opportunities for practice ownership, and that's becoming harder to accomplish. Not to mention the fact that human medicine fields pay better than veterinary ones.

So, all other staff in our office are women, besides the owning veterinarian. And you can bet that's the only person Preacher felt worthy enough to bestow real conversation upon. We'd have complained more about his overt sexism, but it was honestly to our benefit he didn't want to talk to us in any depth. The female relief vet sure wasn't sad to miss him. We did the bare minimum of interactions when he or his family members arrived. As an aside, I'm not one to be jumpy with accusations of misogyny or sexism. Some of that shit's gotten out of hand, but I will freely state Preacher was one that earned the descriptor. More on that in a moment.

His veterinary offenses? Well, he had a multitude. Let's work our way up.

He got himself a big shepherd. Loved him immensely. His pride and joy. That's not the offense. What was obnoxious was his insistence on measuring the dog's growth, week by week. I mean, we offer plenty of clients the use of our clinic scale to check on their puppy's development, or for those monitoring a diet. No appointment needed, if the exam room isn't tied up. No one took advantage of that to the same degree as the Preacher.

There were periods when he brought that dog in with religious regularity to see how much weight he'd had gained. Bearing stats for us of how tall doggo was "at the withers," with each passing week. As if it were a fucking horse. A horse preparing for the big weigh-in before its championship fight. (*Withers* can be applied to a quadruped, I know. Still sounds obnoxious as shit regarding anything other than a horse.) Not that using our scale is such an inherently big deal, but the man possessed zero awareness of timing. His knack for choosing peak busy hours was truly impeccable. I like to think most people have enough perception to read the room and see when it's not an ideal moment. We might be elbow deep in case notes, answering phones, pre-medicating the next surgery patient on the list, refereeing a match in the lobby between families whose pets hate each other, and trying to keep quiet for the euthanasia happening in the exam room, and we could almost guarantee that would be the inopportune moment the door chimed to announce Preacher and his dog, asking to use the exam scale again.

What else?

They left bills unpaid for too long. Charging is now against our clinic's payment policy, and the Preacher's family were one of the prime offenders who brought about that change. (Every facility has its own payment policy, which is usually visibly displayed in the lobby.) It's awkward having to harass anyone for money, week after week, or month after month. It was even more awkward when we had to remind a religious leader that it was coming up to our maximum three-month grace period again, and they still owed us. Not even for very large amounts. Nagging little bits. They would eventually take care of it, but usually when they needed something again, like baths for the stinky little dogs. Funny how that works. Their timing, not ours.

He and the whole family notoriously missed their scheduled appointments. All the damn time. Grooming, health exam, surgery. All of it. Grooming slots are often like gold dust when the weather is hospitable, and it's a shame when an owner doesn't call to cancel or reschedule an appointment they can't make. By the time we can confirm the no-show, it's too late to cold-call someone else to fill the space. It's a disrespectful waste of our groomer's time.

It was a while before we started keeping track of each missed appointment for Preacher and crew. We usually don't bother until one becomes a repeat offender. Grooming was rude, but it was the more expensive missed surgery slots that really started to cross the line. The man put off neutering that big shepherd for a while, wanting to give the dog every opportunity to grow to full potential. He didn't seem keen on the idea, really. Hesitated when it was vaguely "time" to do it and missed the first neuter scheduled. Came by the clinic numerous times to chat with the older male vet about it. Our doctor initially gave his recommendation, but people like Preacher wear you down. When we know someone's not listening or waiting for us to say what they want to hear, we quit trying to convince them. It's not worth our endeavor. The doctor just started giving him that and said, "Sure, you don't have to," because it was easier than a debate.

Veterinary advice wasn't the only thing Preacher wanted from our vet. He seemed to respect him as a wise confidant and sought his opinion on other matters. One time, I overheard Preacher saying he was dissatisfied with the service from another unrelated business and called our vet to rant about it. To get the vet's thoughts on how he should handle the matter. I don't remember what advice was given, but I do recall Preacher said, good man as he was, shouldn't he be bashing the other business with a bad online review? That was the mature way to handle it, right? (This is the part where I weep for humanity.)

Eventually, the family started having problems with the shepherd dog. Aggressive little outbursts towards the other dogs. Go figure. Suddenly that neutering idea came back to the table. Alas, the hesitancy remained. Or maybe it was just their inconsiderate attitude towards other people's time. They made another surgery appointment, and missed it again. And again. And again. Four missed surgical slots made us a little less polite. By the last incident, we were joking amongst ourselves that we could have double-booked the slot and been confident it wouldn't be a problem. Preacher's shepherd wasn't going to show when he was wanted.

Most vet audiences are now wondering why we didn't have a cancellation policy that charges penalties. We should have. No way around that. The only thing I can say is that it was a small clinic in a small town. It's a rare exception for us to keep a client's payment information on file, because we simply didn't have a good method for it. Our veterinary software program didn't store such details, so if we wanted to have it, that data had to be written down and tucked into the client's paper file.

In cases such as Preacher's, enough was enough. The manager and I drafted a letter that was mailed to him and his family. It was firm, to the point, but not rude. It did *not* state we were charging them for any of the already-missed appointments, of which there were many. But it did state our expectation that in future, such a policy would be in place, as far as they were concerned. No-call-no-shows would be penalized with a fee of the equivalent of the exam price. Deposits would be required for a surgery slot. Kind regards, etc. It was signed from the manager of our clinic.

Preacher took it in stride and came to learn to error of his ways.

Just kidding …

Preacher threw a fit when he received that letter. It was at this point we concluded he had memorized the two doctors' differing schedules, to time his outburst during one of the few mornings when the male vet was out of the office. The manager bore the barrage while stationed behind the lobby desk that morning. Preacher came in clutching the letter, shaking it furiously in his fist, and yelling at the woman whose name was signed to it. The relief vet and I were far down the hall, in the middle of a surgery that had the courtesy to show up, but we could hear what we thought was a distant voice raised in anger.

The manager was trembling from the adrenaline of the moment when she came down to surgery to tell us what happened. Preacher had expressed his outrage and left with the threat that she could be sure the owning veterinarian could expect a call from him.

Of course the incident was relayed to the owning vet. I was inwardly, or maybe not-so-inwardly rejoicing—this would be the end of Preacher's tenure as a client.

As promised, Preacher went over her head and spoke with the man he did like, a day or two later. The vet who had approved that ire-inducing letter, as a matter of fact. I was pleased when I could hear snippets of the conversation, in which our vet told the man he agreed with his staff over the problem of our time and money lost, and also clarified that Preacher had been rude to his manager. Secure in that, I went back to my work. Some time later, the vet emerged from his office.

"All taken care of," he happily announced to the manager and me.

A breath of fresh air! "So he's fired?"

The vet shook his head. "No, we talked about it and he's going to be on his best behavior from now on, and …"

The look on my face surely stopped his speech. Best behavior wasn't what we wanted. No apology could be good enough. We wanted him gone. Period.

Alas, Preacher had apparently begged the vet. Pleaded. Implored him for mercy, because he didn't like any other vets in town, and only trusted us. To his credit, our vet hadn't knelt to his complaint about the letter, but he gave in when Preacher asked forgiveness and a second chance. Well, Preacher got his second chance, but the vet was then in the doghouse as far as the manager and I were concerned. Hell, I was the one meaner about it. The manager might have been the one yelled at, but I was the one who raged. Shamed him for not cutting Preacher off there and then, when he deserved it. That wretched man wasn't going to change.

The vet didn't confront or argue back with me. I think he knew he'd let me down and felt guilty. He offered to be the one to deal with Preacher during his appointments. Perhaps I didn't have enough appreciation for the awkward spot he was in at the time. Maybe I could have extended a bit more grace. Problem was, the vet could try, but all the staff knew it was impossible for us not to be involved. The vet knew little about handling front desk operations, so one of us would still have to be involved with future interactions.

For months, the family did try to make good on their promise. Careful on thin ice. They showed up for their appointments. The shepherd finally got neutered. The family was polite and all smiles. Preacher was unbearably over-the-top fake. Schmoozing and oiling as best he knew how. Compliments galore! Trying to be the behavior model so his presence would still be tolerated. If I restrained one of the little dogs for a nail trim by the vet, I was glorified. Nauseatingly so.

"Your *girl* is doing such a fine job!" he would declare to the vet. All of us! What fine work by the help!

It was tempting to vomit and blame the mess on a patient. *Your girl.* My career has been moderate in length, but rest assured, this wasn't 1950.

The suck-up attempts would eventually come to an end, though. Fake people can only be fake for so long. His ultimate dismissal was aided by the global pandemic. That topic gets a chapter of its own, but as it pertained to the ultra-conservative Preacher? Well into the summer months of 2020, it was apparently eating at him that we were performing our duties with the policy of curbside service. He resented that little sign on our front door, declaring that clients were expected to wait in their cars. He was sure we were idiots, feeding into the hysteria of an invented illness. To him, it said everything he needed to know about our beliefs and politics.

Once again, he waited until he knew the owning vet was out of the office. In fact, the vet was out of town entirely, which we suspect Preacher well knew.

This time, the relief vet and I were with the manager behind the desk and got to witness the childish outburst. Ignoring the sign on the door, Preacher stepped inside our lobby. No address to the three of us, other than to launch into his short rant about how we were stupid. So stupid, for still insisting on this curbside nonsense, when no other clinic in town was doing such a thing. (Not true.) Our policy was socialist paranoia and we sheep should be ashamed of ourselves!

He should have been ashamed he didn't stay long enough to get an earful from us. But, coward that he was, he darted back outside as quickly as he'd come in to insult us. Our jaws had collectively dropped from that unannounced drive-by, but it was the relief vet who spoke first.

"Alright. He's *done*."

We got an eyeful of what he surely thought was a victorious departure. He climbed back into his off-roading probably-not-street-legal vehicle. Devoted wife at his side. Dog overflowing from the back. Politically charged flags billowing proudly in the wind from either side of the bed, informing anyone in sight how he felt.

This time, Preacher was unequivocally fired as a client.

A very brief letter was mailed. This time, stating it would be for the best of everyone if they took their business elsewhere. Pet records were enclosed. No further need to contact our clinic.

There was a final contact from Preacher, privately messaged to the owner vet's social media account. Of course, we all got a chance to read it, too. Just to marvel at the level of insanity we'd had on our hands for all that time.

In all its glory, this two-paragraph diatribe began with a rather jovial, "Greetings." The remainder of the onslaught was a trainwreck of crimes against grammar, skewed claims about the final event, and demeaning political accusations. A nonsensical rambling of how the boss had allowed himself to be corrupted by the staff's wicked agenda. How we hated our country. How we wretched ones refused to pass on his gift of a certain partisan-themed hat to the vet. Perhaps the *magnum opus* was his saintly insistence that he was never rude to our "Socialist baby killing employee." Seems relevant to report that presumptive label was mentioned no less than three times. This impressive piece of work was rounded off with the notion that we, *the socialists*, were the ones suffering from the loss of him.

Oh, Bless his heart.

We appreciated his valuable feedback and aimed to do bett—Nah. Fuck that guy.

No response was ever given. I mean, what was the point? Nearly every statement in the message was flawed. No need to prolong a conversation with such ridiculous accusations and outright lies, start to finish. Where would we begin? A man that assumed our politics by a sign on the door for curbside service isn't someone we needed to keep on. To my knowledge, no employee had ever had a conversation with him about the joys of abortion. Or any political leaning. We also never saw the gift in question. For the record, had Preacher offered it nicely, we would have placed the item on the doctor's desk. The vet wouldn't have worn it, but we'd still have offered it.

But with that conclusion, the Socialist baby-ki—I mean, the *manager* and I, were glad to wipe our hands of Preacher and his family. As a business, we strive to be respectful of anyone's creed, as it's usually *none of our business*.

Please, don't make it our business.

Running Interference

"The most important thing to do in your life is to not interfere with somebody else's life."
—Frank Zappa

Strictly speaking, my objective at work is to promote the health of pets. I don't ask to know details about the lives of the humans that own them. That said, inevitably when taking patient history, such information comes out. Or is willingly spilled. Sometimes it does become relevant in identifying the diagnosis of the pet, or it affects the treatment plan. When that personal sharing happens, I tailor my questions to be as non-invasive as possible. Privacy is a right. It's a delicate balance, having those honest and open discussions about the environment of the pet.

With most of our married clients, we often only see one of the spouses for appointments. A designated partner handles the bulk of the vet visits. It's fine for us to have continuity between our communications. In some cases, I've never seen the other spouse for all the years of their pet's care, until it's time for the end-of-life discussion.

This isn't a euthanasia story, though. This is an upset in communication.

In this instance, it was the wife who always brought the dog in. A shepherd-cattle dog mix. Anyone who knows those breeds well knows they can be a challenge. Often, they bond to a single person and are protective of them, but don't care to open up to others. Prone to dramatics, territorial, anxious and willing to snap when they're uncomfortable about a situation. Her dog thankfully didn't give us too much trouble, but he still had his temperamental moments. We'll call him Bingo. We'd learned his personality quirks through the years and could identify what Bingo was touchy about. Knowing he was anxious, she usually dragged him straight through the lobby door and into the exam room, and when it was done, she'd drag him directly to the car to wait while she came back inside to pay and receive her prescriptions. No chance for a canine meltdown in the lobby. Common sense, and I always appreciated that about her.

One fateful day, we received a call. Not from her, but from her husband. Apparently, she had had to go out of town for a week or so, and while she was gone, Bingo had gotten himself into a small scrape. Details were vague. A minor puncture wound on Bingo's chest. Bingo was a country dog—a hairy one, at that—and might have run into anything.

The husband didn't ask to bring Bingo in, but inquired about what he should do. The office manager was the one taking the call, and through some careful questioning, got the gist of it. Husband couldn't quite see the wound through the matted hair, so he wasn't sure how serious it was. Shallow, deep, small, extensive, who knew? The obvious suggestion was that he should bring Bingo in for an exam. He was offered rapid appointment times, but hem-hawed over that, apparently uncomfortable about handling the dog. It was the wife's dog, he said, and he had a hard time getting near him. The matter was discussed over more than one phone call.

I believe the husband did tell the wife about the wound while she was gone.

As our manager tried to offer the husband helpful suggestions for how it might be managed to bring Bingo in, he laid it out.

"The dog hates me, and the feeling's mutual."

The amount of time it took him to say it made it clear it was a sensitive point.

Well, that was that. We couldn't force him to bring Bingo in, nor in good conscience, recommend he try to treat the mystery wound with any home first aid. If Bingo injured him in the process, it would only be too easy for him to blame us for the advice. That whole liability thing.

All we could do was have him watch and wait, and if the wound wasn't healing on its own, it was certain the wife would bring the dog in anyways, once she got home from her trip. At least it didn't sound like Bingo was in immediate danger.

Well, lo and behold, when the wife came home, we got an irritated phone call. Precious Bingo had an injury, and why hadn't we seen him for an exam days before? We were stunned. By her accusations, it didn't take long for us to figure out the husband had lied to her about the nature of our communications. He led her to believe he'd done the right thing in calling for an appointment, but we'd blown him off. Uncaringly dismissing Bingo's wound for days.

In a delicate way, the office manager tried to smooth things over and offered for her to come in with the dog right away. The wife was obviously still mad, but she did come. She wouldn't let her immediate feelings get in the way of the treatment the dog needed. Now, our manager is a person who does not care for confrontation, so she made herself absent during the appointment time. She and the doctor were still trying to determine how to handle it.

I helped see Bingo during his exam. He had a shallow wound that was cleaned up and treated with antibiotics. Nothing terribly serious, but we certainly didn't want it to get infected. The wife let me know when she checked out, she appreciated the veterinarian's care, as she always had. However, she was *not* happy with the service at the desk, and she wanted to hear an apology from the manager. Or an acknowledgment. An explanation. Something.

It wasn't necessarily my place to jump into the middle of it. Put on the spot, I could only softly suggest I had been under the impression her husband had been offered an appointment. I was too stubborn to apologize for something that wasn't our fault. It was clear she didn't believe that. She left. I passed on the awkward message.

It was a delicate situation, though I do wish we'd handled it differently. The vet and the manager discussed it several times over the next couple of days, mutually tending to agree with each other they ought to leave it alone. Neither wanted to insert themselves between a married couple and stir up drama. How is a business supposed to tell a wife her husband is a liar? That it wasn't our fault?

Without divulging private information, I told my own husband about the scenario.

"You should absolutely tell her," he said. "It's not about coming between them, but about the patient in your care and how you responded to it. It involves the clinic."

Well, he had a point. It was our reputation and maybe we deserved to be able to defend ourselves against the suggestion we ignored a patient. Marital strife be damned. I brought that up with my fellow staff, but in the end, it didn't happen. The manager stuck with not interfering. Putting off the phone call that was giving her anxiety.

The wife came back to the clinic a few days after her appointment. She asked for Bingo's medical records. Angry and disappointed that, in her mind, she'd not been made priority enough to warrant a courtesy call. She'd given us a fair amount of time and gotten no response. It's not as though I could blame her for that perspective, though I badly wanted to tell her the truth. That our staff were sweating and frustrated over the incident, the manager had probably lost sleep over it, and oh yeah, your husband is a fucking liar about what happened to make himself look good while throwing us under the bus. But I didn't say any of that. I could only say I understood her position as I made the requested copies to transfer to another clinic.

We never saw her again. I can only hope the husband felt some measure of guilt for his role, but I'll never know.

Sometimes a situation falls into your lap where you do feel compelled to interfere, in thinking about what consequences people will live with when it's over.

Pets get hit by cars every day. It's the responsibility of an owner to keep their animal contained, safe, or well-trained enough to avoid a road. Of course, accidents happen. However, my small town was notorious for roaming dogs and no one enforcing leash laws.

One such case rushed into the clinic while we were on the last appointment of the day. I encountered the panicked young man in the lobby, lugging an unconscious Doberman-mix in his arms, followed by two women and a girl. With the exam room occupied, I cleared a space on our lobby table for pending prescriptions. He laid down the limp dog for my quick assessment and attempt at CPR, which has a poor success rate in dogs.

Dead on arrival.

I knew it already, but for their sake, snuck quickly into the exam room to grab my stethoscope to be sure, murmuring to the vet that I would need him in short order to confirm. I checked all signs and vitals before telling them I was sorry, but their dog had already passed. The expected tears ensued. The women and little girl petted the newly deceased dog through their wailing and then collapsed themselves on the lobby bench to process.

It didn't take long to piece together what happened. The young man was not part of the family of women, but was the driver who hit the dog while going home through his neighborhood. The dog had jumped out in front of his truck. Simple as that.

"If we'd gotten here sooner, would she still be alive?" the little girl boldly asked me.

They'd come as soon as it had happened. Couldn't have taken more than five or so minutes to arrive at our facility. Small town.

"No, sweetheart. She wouldn't," I said firmly.

Given the condition of the dog, I thought my answer to be well within *reasonable* medical probability. It was highly unlikely two or three minutes would have mattered. Could I have said that with a hundred-percent certainty? Nah. I couldn't. I don't possess an omniscient answer. But what would be the purpose of conveying any miniscule doubt to a child, who would forever be traumatized by the day her dog got hit on the road? She didn't need to hear that. She needed certainty. That, despite their efforts to act quickly, it wasn't possible to save her pet.

Eventually the family asked what to do with the body. We gently presented burial and cremation quotes.

While they weighed those options, I looked at the driver again.

Pale. Speechless. In shock, and unable to bear looking at the heartbroken family. His gaze was fixed forward at the reception counter. Emotion welling to the surface, doing everything he could to swallow it. I stood before him, leaning in to quietly address him alone.

"It's not your fault," I said. "It could have happened to anyone. But it is *not* your fault, ok?"

The driver's lip quivered. He couldn't answer me, too internally distraught. I knew he'd still go home, wracked with guilt and haunted by the little girl's tears. He was a decent person doing the best he could. Wordlessly, he paid for their selected cremation.

He'd feel remorse, no matter what I said. Still, I hoped that once the shock wore off, that he'd take it to heart. I meant it. As I saw it, the driver wasn't to blame.

A hard lesson. Of course, I didn't voice the harsh truth aloud amidst everyone's devastation in that lobby. I just hoped they learned for the next pet.

For the Sake of Levity: Something's Afoot

I debated whether to file this as comic relief, or to try mentioning it as a more serious retelling. Frankly, as awful as it is, I can't *not* still laugh about it.

The hospital offered the service of dropping off your pet in the morning, if committing to a mid-day appointed timeslot was inconvenient. Usually this was an easy method for annual preventive care exams, updating vaccines and such. Less frequently was this used for sick cases. Then, staff worked your pet in during the day when there were free moments between the scheduled appointments.

One of our clients opted for the drop-off route on this otherwise ordinary morning. At the lobby desk, she confirmed the items her dachshund-mix needed to be caught up, then passed the sweet little pooch over the counter to the receptionist.

"Oh, by the way," she said, before turning to go. "The foot fell off. I'll be back for him after 5:00. Bye!"

The stunned receptionist processed that information, and then saw for herself that indeed, there was an appendage missing. She stuttered a moment, calling after the client in a desperate bid for more information. What the …? Why …?

How …?

Apparently, the dog had had some terrible injury, of what nature I couldn't tell you. But the wound had caused his leg to be nearly severed at the hock joint. They opted to let nature take its course, and whether the dog chewed off the remaining end of his hind leg or it finally rotted away on its own, there sure as fuck wasn't a foot where a foot ought to have been. The amazing part was the owner had only brought the dog to catch up on preventive care. She had zero concern about the unorthodox amputation. The event just so happened to closely coincide with his annual exam.

It's the first and last time I can say the whiteboard listing of a patient's To-Do checklist and points of concern contained the words, "foot, fell off." And yes, we laughed about it all day long. A new genre of jokes in which the punchline revolved around limbs overtaken by gravity. Niche market, that line of comedy.

Examining the remains of the joint, it was still recent enough that we thought we could help the situation. Our very by-the-book vet called the owner with her extensive recommendations. Owner was annoyed. Balking, insistent her dog was fine. She gave in only to the bare minimum injection of an antibiotic, "If you think it's *absolutely* necessary."

"I do," the vet said.

The Lewd, The Rude, The Less-Than-Shrewd

"Difficult people are the greatest teachers."
—Pema Chodron

Let's be transparent. This chapter is a shameless placement for nothing more than sharing a few stories of encountering less-than-ideal clientele. I present them in no particular order.

The Lewd

I don't expect to get hit on at work.

If I awkwardly have to rate myself, I guess I'm tolerable and have received flirtations a fair number of times in my life. However, flirtation has little place in a veterinary clinic. Not many single guys (or gals) are strolling through my hospital lobby looking for love from a veterinary technician. Maybe when I get around to writing the SOAP Opera book ...

Now, back in my bartending days at the local pub? Yes. That's the setting. I supply the order of booze, and while I'm trapped behind the bar and the imbiber's inhibitions get lower and lower, that's the time I expect to hear what a purty mouth I have. To dodge grabby hands. Or find digits left behind for me on a soggy coaster.

But in a medical facility? Nah. Not the vibe. Besides. The alcohol in this building is 70% isopropyl. Wouldn't recommend it.

When romantic pursuit does happen at the clinic, it's a rare occasion. And thankfully more subtle than the pub. Usually. Someone lingering too long at the desk at check-out, for example. Finding extra things to chat about. I mean, everyone likes to gab with us about their pet and funny things they do. We hear it all day long, and while it's often an easy social lubricant for socially awkward people like us animal-lovers, we do sometimes tire of being interested in the ad nauseum anecdotes. In one gentleman's case, it just went beyond the average expected time to tell me about his cute bottle-feeder kittens.

Sometimes we'd reach to the back of the desk for our personal phones, subtly calling our own front desk line to suddenly appear busy, needing to take that oh-so-important call. Or if you were sympathetic enough to your coworker in the same scenario, you might call from the back room, pretending to have a long-winded question. My office manager nearly lost her composure when I impersonated a shopping client, asking for every single price-point of every preventive parasite product on the shelf, and their corresponding deals.

The more overt flirts? I don't know what it is, but I tend to attract men many years my senior. Not that I don't appreciate a silver fox. I do. But within reason. In this particular client's case, he could have been my grandfather. My frail grandfather, whose dog needed to have a stool sample checked. Given the client's limited mobility, I politely offered to jog doggo outside, choosing our own clinic-provided leash, rather than the *Service Dog* harness the poorly-kempt, reeking-of-cigarettes patient definitely hadn't earned. What a mood-setting buzzkill, right? Did our thing. Mission successful, doggo and I made our way back to the building with our collected sample. As I walked past the client to get back into the building, he felt that would be the choice moment to tell me what a fine job I did. And how fine a day it would be if he scored my phone number …

It's the first and only time I've been holding a literal shitbag and been hit on.

I hate to crush all your hopes for the rom-com meet-cute, but alas. He did not score my number, and I doubt we'll see that plot point in the upcoming holiday movie season.

The other, eh, incident which comes to mind? I'd like to say it was accidental, but I do know I was mortified. When you restrain animals for a living, there's not much room for personal space. You accept it as part of the job. Your coworker's butt is going to end up in your face, and you'll return the favor at some point, because it just makes sense in X-scenario to hold the dog that way. Shower and deodorize for their sake, please. What I don't accept very well is having my space violated by the client.

To be fair, the exam room was quite small. I stood alongside the client while the doctor was stationed on the opposite side of the table. Client was a big man. In the kindest terms, he possessed a rather large gut. And while I held his cat for the examination, he decided he would be more helpful standing on the other side of the table, where nervous kitty could see him better. In that room, there was very little space to move past me. Didn't deter him. No problem. Suddenly his hand felt its way along the small of my back for guidance as he made his move. And the next thing I knew, I was practically bent over the exam table.

By a gut. A massive gut, pressing me over by the waist. Taking its time to shuffle past.

The veterinarian couldn't contain his laughter but tried to play it off as playful chatter with the patient. Surely enjoying the pure horror on my face while I tried to pretend it wasn't happening.

I'm not sure what base we reached there, but my supervising vet couldn't wait to tell all the other staff about the humiliating moment at my expense.

Coworkers have had their run-ins, too. I worked for a stunning veterinarian once. I recall walking past and seeing a client practically serenading her out in the lobby, while she turned tomato-red. Shocked that such a beauty could have been the one providing care for his pets, rather than some crusty-looking scientist, he tried impressing her with his enormous wealth. Could have backed it up, too.

An older male veterinarian has a trio of middle-to-later-aged ladies we tease him about. One you'll find mention of in another Levity bit, with her dog in need of having anal glands expressed. She has no problem flagrantly flirting with the vet, in front of her own husband. There was an infamous incident where she brought an out-of-town friend on a Hot Doctors Tour of our town, which included our guy. The second admirer bakes for him and ensures she has numerous appointments for her pets scattered about as often as she can. Vaccine schedules spread all over the place. Shave the matted hair off the cat another day. Come by to buy flea and tick product separately, just so she can visit more frequently to chat about her favorite topics with him. She brings written lists sometimes. The majority of those topics are innocent enough, but she does have a strange obsession with bringing up her annual pap smears. Maybe it's meant to be seductive. And the third, probably most attractive, of the three fans—er, clients—strikes me as the rich housewife. Bit bored. She might bake him a birthday cake, or flaunt herself in his direction if the occasion could possibly permit. He doesn't hate it when he gets a hug.

One older woman was decidedly comfortable in her own skin. In the exam room, her little dog was precariously tucked inside her baggy shirt, in indecent-to-reach places. When the vet arrived and saw the half-undressing act underway to pull the dog out, he elected to do the professional thing, tactfully stepping back out of the room until she was decent, and the dog was freed. He thought he was being a courteous gentleman, but when he returned, that lady client gave him an indignant earful for having left. "What does it even *matter*, Doctor? *I'm* comfortable!" she ranted, oddly insistent that he should have stayed.

Has it ever crossed a line? The most egregious incident happened fairly recently to a fellow staff member. She's known this client for years, in the context of him being a married man. A mildly strange person, but seemingly harmless. A few months ago, his wife passed, which we learned about in our small-town news. Shortly after, the weird commentary began.

His primary business with our clinic had been grooming appointments for his small dog. He said little to any other staff members, but when the object of his interest was alone at the desk, he started hinting to her. Nothing of the typical fashion to suggest he was trying to flirt. Instead, he made insinuations about her past. One day, it was a comment that he remembered her as a prominent party-girl at the bars when they were younger. That resulted in her giving him a quizzical look, and boldly stating that if he claimed that, *he* must have been the one frequenting those establishments, because she was hardly ever that girl at the bar. She would freely tell me as an aside that while she had had fun in youth, there was no way our client ran in the same circles. The age gap between them would have been a creepy non-starter, "back in the day."

We wondered if he was remembering another woman of similar looks, but he seemed so sure of it and had been so stealthy in the manner in which he delivered that information, so as to unnerve her. Avoiding the other staff, finding close proximity, and speaking it in hushed tones. Like an accusation of some filthy past. Like it was their dirty secret.

The next time, it escalated. When he managed to catch her alone again at checkout, they finished the grooming transaction. Then he leaned over the counter to speak in a lower tone.

"I have pictures of you," he told her.

"Excuse me?" she retorted.

"Nothing. Never mind," he decided.

Perturbed, and rightly so, she tried to press him to clarify his statement. He refused to explain his incredibly creepy comment and left immediately after.

We discussed it at length when she told the rest of us. There was no confusing it with an innocuous statement such as, "Oh, I found an old yearbook photo of you the other day!" No. Nothing like that. It was absolutely, without a doubt, a creepy-as-fuck, seedy accusation for which there was no plausible explanation. I wouldn't have been surprised to learn he found out where she lived and took peeping photos.

The next time he calls for an appointment, he's going to be told he's not welcome back for being inappropriate towards staff. I do so look forward to that.

Unlike the pub-setting, flirtatious occasions don't happen often for us, so when it does, it tends to be a notable event. Does it ever happen the other way around, you may wonder? Maybe you didn't wonder, but you'll have my answer anyways.

I've never heard a fellow staff member blatantly hit on a client. That I was aware of. If they had, they likely wouldn't have lasted long in their employment, because it's wildly inappropriate. At least within the context of the veterinary premises. There's a but, of course, because there's always a "but." But … we're humans, too. Sure, we notice when a client is attractive. We try not to make a big thing of it, treat them the same as the next, but I'd be a liar if I said my coworkers didn't occasionally get excited when a certain client was on the day's schedule. Passing the word along to the others, to check their hair in the bathroom, or whatever professional courtesy. Good old team spirit. Hey, you gotta trust your medical team. Have each others' backs.

One morning, I needed the microchip scanner to confirm placement in my post-op surgery patient but forgot to take it to the surgical suite. It wasn't on its usual hanger in the exam room, so I figured the receptionist had borrowed it and left it someplace. I sought her out. However, she was nowhere to be found, either. It was a few minutes before she returned, after hanging out the front door of the clinic, microchip scanner in hand.

Apparently, a decent looking gent had found a stray cat and wanted to check for a chip. His foreign accent had kept her hooked, and she'd extended that conversation as long as possible, taking the scanner with her, in the process.

There was a standout husband-and-wife client couple who were *gorgeous*. I'll be honest, I remember nothing else about them. Let's just call them Mr. and Mrs. Jones. They're not my favorites as people or anything, because as I've admitted, I don't remember. Just the superficial gift of being easy on the eyes. No one could deny it, and all the staff were on board with that objective fact. The moment I loved so well was that even my otherwise upstanding-in-professional-dignity supervising veterinarian got excited about seeing their pet on the schedule. He hadn't missed the appeal of Mrs. Jones any more than I missed the optics of Mr. Jones. The vet nudged my arm suggestively.

"A little something for me, and a little something for you!"

The Rude

Anyone who's ever worked in the public service industry knows rude people happen. The veterinary field is no exception. No stranger to the fact. The day-to-day stressors that all humans endure are sometimes enough on their own to instigate unpleasant interactions. Add in the complexity of strong emotions and opinions on one's pet, and it can get nastier.

Sometimes it starts as soon as the client walks in the door. They don't appreciate the verbal request, or the signage asking for their loose pet to be leashed or contained in a carrier. Offended, because their precious darling is well-behaved and they have control over them. One client kept his dog leashed but gave him free reign to go wherever he wanted. Following doggo behind the desk or down the hall to Employee Only designated areas? Sure, be our guest!

It shouldn't be that hard a concept, but some people throw a fit. Your pet may win awards for a sunny disposition, but you know nothing about the other patients in the lobby or coming out of the exam. I have refereed several almost-assaults between animals whose owners were too oblivious to pull their leashed creature away from the other. One client brought her pair of cats properly in a carrier, but set it on the floor during check-in. They used to be pleasant cats in the clinic, but the curious golden retriever, sweet as could be, didn't do them any favors when she wanted to say hello. Kitties were traumatized, and we've dealt with it forever since, at their every visit.

When I was a complete newbie, I worked for the corporate clinic that wanted me to promote our preventive care packages. That whole sales aspect I despise.

It was also a high-volume clinic, and most clients could expect to wait the average amount of time before the veterinarian came in to do their part. In the interim, the lucky bastards got me to fill the time, trying to gather all the patient history, prep materials, impart any client education I could. And then sometimes I'd be trying to fill time. And more time. The vet was taking forever to get out of the adjacent room. I'd poke my head back in and give my client a progress update if I could. Promising the doctor was coming soon.

In this particular case, the client was a "rabies only." By the way, if you're a client that wants rabies vaccination only and decline every other wellness service for your pet, you're absolutely seen as the bottom-dweller. Someone doing the bare minimum. There are rare exceptions for that being tolerable, but most of the time, we're not too impressed by you.

Well, Rabies-Only just wanted the rabies, only. A quick jab for the dog to make him street-legal, pay the incremental fee, and be on his merry way. That wasn't quite working out for him, because my veterinarian was behind schedule. She could tell I was anxiously dancing around, waiting for her to do my quick appointment, but her simultaneous case was more involved. She pushed me off with instructions to go try to promote other services we could offer him in the meantime. More time-filling.

I had already done that. Begrudgingly, I went back and did it again. Obediently following orders. Let's just say he wasn't terribly impressed by whatever pathetic presentation I'd come up with. The subtle giveaway to his feelings had something to do with his screaming, "Jesus Christ, lady! What the hell's taking so long?! Just poke him in the butt and let's go!"

I was too young and nervous then to have had the confidence to stand up for myself. To tell the asshole I was doing my job the best I could. I finally went to the back treatment area and barely kept my seething under control as the vet tried once more to hold me at bay, suggesting what I could do next to occupy more time.

"I can't go back in there. He's ... *yelling* at me."

She could hear it in my voice. Finally, she paused her more urgent case and went to my patient's room. I got the hell out as soon as I wasn't needed, but I was gratified to overhear the vet's skill at motherly scolding in a way that put people in their place. Firmly, but not impolite. Letting him know it wasn't ok to yell at her support staff the way he did.

Years into my career later, I laughed much more over a rabies-only request I got over the phone. By then, more confident and assertive in my role, timidity about defending our clinic's services was no longer a problem for me. Which was helpful when this man wanted the vaccine for his dog, but no other part of the veterinary experience. Nothing. Nada. Zip.

I presumed part of his hesitation (ahem, stubbornness) was concern over the cost. But the veterinarian who was *prospectively* going to perform the injection has the philosophy that rabies-only clients get what they pay for. A cursory look to establish the animal is sound. Then, you guessed it. Rabies, only. He's not going to spend any extra time on a comprehensive exam unless they pay for it. I even tried to explain that to this gentleman, in a delicate way. How we wouldn't be charging extra for a full exam. He still wasn't having it.

"Look, I just want him to come out into the parking lot, and I've got the dog in my truck. Don't even look at him. Just give him the shot and I'll give you the money. That's it. Don't want none of your paperwork or nothing like th—"

"Sir, it doesn't work like that," I tried for the fourth time. Attempting to carefully lay out the concept that we don't do exams in vehicles except under very special circumstances. Safety protocols and restraint, blah, blah. How there wouldn't be an exam fee. Even if we weren't doing a full exam, that we sort of, kind of, maybe, have to at least lay eyes upon the dog. Silly preference on our part to avoid accidentally poking doggo in the eye. He was oddly insistent on that part, though. Not looking at his dog. I half expected him to ask us to be blindfolded. And forget the explanation about the Rabies Certificate. He didn't want to create a damn account! No need for names and addresses and paper and …

I couldn't help but think he must have been ordered by some entity to have his dog vaccinated. Seems a bit odd he wouldn't want the certificate to prove it. Nonsensical. That's what most people want.

Not our special guy, though. The phone call ended with him in a fury because I wouldn't comply with his weird-ass request. I think I got the final word of saying, "We're not going to do that. You could try elsewh—" before he hung up on me.

I wonder how he's doing, sometimes.

Others are willing to put a little bit more money into their pet exams. But they may come with a preconceived notion of what they want done. Playing doctor themselves, is how I think of it. I despise that. This isn't Burger King, ma'am. You don't get to have it your way. This is medicine.

One such lady was used to the treatment plan for her cat's chronic conditions with her regular veterinarian and knew what she wanted. When she was landed with the relief vet one day, who had different ideas after the cat's exam, the lady threw a childish fit and stormed out of the clinic. Bitching about the injustice of not getting her way.

Another gal brought her dog into our hospital for a persistent cough. She knew what she wanted when she arrived. Cough medicine. Cut and dry. She'd diagnosed it herself. Just needed us to give her the goods.

Alas, the vet actually did his exam anyways, as good vets are wont to do. Felt the need to recommend diagnostics to rule out other more sinister origins to the symptoms, besides only treating the symptom itself. He gave me his proposed treatment plan for the patient. It was my job to present that treatment plan to the client for approval. If she declined, to clarify her concerns and help formulate Plan B. I scanned the items before going back into that room. Exam, radiographs, and an estimate for potential therapies based on the interpretation of the proposed radiographs. That sort of thing. Pretty standard.

Client didn't think so. From her reaction, I might as well have walked in and kicked her in the face.

"What the hell is this?" she screamed. "X-rays? Are you kidding me? You want me to pay for X-rays for a *cough*?! What the—Oh my God. Get this shit out of here and just give me the damn cough tablets!"

Years later, I wish I'd seen that lady in the clinic where I would have been allowed to tell her to fuck off for being so rude. Alas, since it was frowned upon at that particular place of employment, I begged for any other VA or VT to be the one to finish the discharge. None was available. I was saddled with that peach.

I didn't have the authority to say what I wanted to Her Hatefulness, but I didn't have to be polite at that point, either. I flung her prescription on the exam table, told her to read the directions, and to check out with the front desk. She seemed surprised I wasn't kissing her ass.

While that incident is the more common scenario, of clients rejecting a treatment option due to cost, or even disbelief in the recommendation, I recently saw the rare opposite in a case.

Our tenure with this client was painfully short. The youngish woman called one morning to start a new account with us. Her pitbull had sarcoptic mange, she claimed.

I knew right away she was either in some medical field, or the kind of person who had spent time researching, because while most people have heard of mange itself, few add the "sarcoptic" specification. She did. I had doubts as to whether it would be a true mange case. For as often as I hear clients throw the word around, it's seldom, truly, mange, a skin disease caused by mites hanging out in hair follicles, which causes a myriad of symptoms such as itching, hair loss, redness, oozing, and crusty lesions. Severe cases can affect appetite and energy level. Still, I listened patiently as she confirmed my suspicion. Relaying she had spent months researching and applying over-the-counter remedies to the poor dog. But by then—and at this point, her voice was starting to break with the effort of restraining emotion—she felt she was at a loss. The dog wasn't getting better, only worse. In fact, now it was dire and the poor thing was really suffering. Despite all her valiant attempts. She cried as she explained the problem had become more than what she could handle, and it was time to accept she needed help.

I hate to make assumptions about people before meeting them in person, but I had a strong feeling this was an unstable person. Months of home and OTC remedies were worthless, and only now it was dire? The phrasing of her words led me to believe she was more upset at her perceived failure in her attempts at healing than the actual suffering of the dog. I felt sorry for the animal before it even showed up. Expecting it would be so riddled with a skin condition that its quality of life was diminished, or even on death's door, the way she cried.

I prepared her for the cost of the exam to start, which she agreed to. Then made her a quick appointment for later that same morning, out of concern for the new patient.

When she arrived, I peeked over the lobby counter to see what disgraceful situation was going to be tied to the other end of the leash. I looked at the dog. And then at my schedule. Looked at the dog in front of the counter again, and mentally confirmed the clock read the time I thought it was.

Yep, that was her.

Dog looked back at me. Tail wagging pleasantly. Perked ears. Eyes bright and alert. Coat clean and free of any blemishes. I watched them follow one of my assistants into the exam room.

"So ... I sort of expected it to look like a leper, the way that lady was crying on the phone," I whispered to the manager, after they were out of earshot.

"Right?" she agreed. "That dog looks perfectly healthy!"

Still, didn't want to fully assume. Maybe it had a ventrum full of sores I couldn't see at a quick glance, or something. Shrugging it off for the moment, the manager and I diverted our attention to a product order. We'd ask the assistant how the appointment went when it was over.

Well, we caught the tail end as the client was leaving the exam room, tension deep in her voice.

"So, you don't like pitbulls?" she said accusatorily toward the veterinarian.

The manager and I stopped chatting, too curious to overhear. And once again, a paraphrased version of the same.

"So, you have a problem with pitbulls."

Manager and I were immediately concerned the appointment hadn't gone well. We hadn't heard any commotion, but perhaps the dog had snapped or been poorly behaved. Maybe the client didn't like seeing her dog restrained. Shortly after, she was gone. When we emerged to ask the VA what the hell happened, she filled us in.

Client had talked over the doctor constantly. Interrupting him with her opinions and hardly listening to his medical observations. The dog was perfectly well-behaved. Sat on the table nicely. No problems there. But when the doctor stated that for her breed, the dog's skin looked great, with no signs of mange or any other concerning dermal lesions, client wasn't having it. She'd convinced herself the dog was ill. That it was in devastating shape. No amount of reassurance from the veterinarian (the one with the medical degree) could persuade her otherwise. And she didn't care for his phrasing of, "For a pitbull, she's got good skin. A lot of them have skin issues, but she looks good today."

As a gesture of goodwill, he offered her a basic course of antibiotics for the dog, if it would make her feel better. She said it would. But then couldn't let go the notion her opinion or her dog's breed had been slighted.

Client had then taken the DVM's medical observation about breed tendencies and twisted his words to play some sort of wronged-victim card. Thus, the accusation we'd heard. That our vet didn't like pitbulls. She stood there in our lobby crying at the perceived insult to her pet. Decided she wasn't going to wait for the VA to finish putting the prescription label on her pills, or to check out at the desk.

"Fuck you guys," she decided, and stormed out. Without pills, nor payment.

To be honest, that one doesn't make me angry. Clearly there's a mental health issue unresolved in that woman's world, and I doubt she would have been happy at all, unless we'd gone along with her own assessment and racked up an unnecessary bill for mange treatment.

But she brings up another pet peeve of mine. (Ha! *Pet* peeve, because this is a veterinary b—never mind.)

People who like to talk without listening. That might have even been mentioned before. Good listeners are worth their weight in gold. We have several clients who like to ask questions, but don't take a breath long enough to hear the answer. Instead, they ramble on through your every attempt of "Yes, so we can—er—- no, that's not a prob—yes—well, based on today's exam, we th—oh, yes. Sure. Uh-huh."

If you don't shut the fuck up to hear the answer, I'm not going to bother.

One of our worst offenders was an elderly man we honestly only still tolerate because of his wife. She's aware he's an ass and goes out of her way to apologize for it and smooth things over. We're not dumb. We see that. We know why the groomer got a huge tip. Or why he finally came in but sat on the bench and didn't say a word. Because she finally threatened him out in the car beforehand to keep his damn mouth shut and not start something.

He would come in and ask questions but talk over every attempt to answer. Why was the dog having such a problem with her anal glands? What did her weight have to do with anything? Did we hold her down and rip the excess hair out of her ears like he asked, and cut the nails to bleeding-short, or was he going to be upset?

He was going to be upset, I'm sure. Our vet wasn't going to be bullied into mistreating his dog.

The most egregious fact we learned about this client was that he, himself, was a veterinarian. And never bothered to divulge this information until he'd been bringing his pets to us for well over a year. Spent all that time presumably "testing" us to see if we measured up to whatever his personal standards were. Not that he ever paused long enough to let us give the full answer to his question. At first, we thought he was lying about his credentials, but later looked him up, and sure enough. Licensed Vet. Not sure what area of work he chose, but it's hard to imagine he ever worked in practice from how rude and argumentative he was.

At one point, we pissed him off because we wouldn't send home a rabies vaccine for him to give the dogs himself. A vet should know better on that no-no. A rabies vaccine has to be administered by a vet *employed by the premises* providing the vaccine, and is recorded under a specific vet's license number, or premises. Lot of legalities attached to it. We don't just go giving those out.

Someone with medical credentials to their name should be held to a higher standard. Not be the one asking for the cutting-corner deals that interfere with medical ethics.

That note brings me to the last rudeness subject. Human nurses.

God bless you for what you do, human nurses. Truly. Wholly. You earn all the praise for the shit you put up with, and I admit I could not do the job you do. My own family has several members of your club, and I love them dearly.

But when it comes to veterinary medicine? Stay the fuck in your lane. There are similarities sometimes, yes. You can draw on those comparisons if it helps you to care for your own pet. However, there are differences in our professional recommendations we ask you to respect, because … well, we're working on entirely different species. Keep that in the forefront of your mind.

Nurses have been some of the outright rudest clients I've witnessed, and it's a fucking shame to say. They think they know better than us about the job we do every day.

I once worked a shift alongside a VA who was almost on the verge of tears because of her client, and she asked if I could finish the appointment for her. The lady was a nurse, and without any other introduction, looked at our staff member's name tag and title, and basically berated her for not being good enough for the role. Lecturing the VA on her own worthiness as a credentialed nurse, and if our VA wanted to ever amount to anything more than worthless, ought to get herself into a program to redeem herself. The language I'm using here isn't far off from what she said to our poor VA. She hadn't bothered to even have a conversation with her first. To ask about educational pursuits, career goals, or any such thing. Just made a dickish assumption about a person she didn't know and hatefully criticized her for it.

I took over the room and found her every bit as awful as the VA promised. She started to demand the same of me. I snapped at her that I was in VT school (which was true at the time), and the vet and I were pretty cold in our reception of her. She tried to explain herself to us, and we just let the rudeness hang there in the air. Unanswered. Unacknowledged, because it didn't deserve the justification she tried to give to it. We finished the necessary items for her pet and sent her on her vile way.

Others have been known to argue with staff when we recommend services, because they "know" it's not really necessary, and we're just upcharging our shit. Heartworm test? Please. We don't need that money-grab. Screw you for recommending it to me.

As an aside, I once had a non-nurse lady call to ask what services to expect for her dog's annual exam. When I mentioned a heartworm check, she told me she'd had dogs her whole life (which makes her an authority) and had never heard of such a thing as a heartworm. She then accused me of making it up as some conspiracy to get her money. "Grab 'em and stab 'em!" one of my vets likes to joke … I mean, I wish I were that good, but regretfully, I don't possess the talent to come up with a scheme on that level, nor do I have control of some horde of mosquitos to spread my dastardly plan. But if I had, why am I not personally reaping the profits from this lucrative business? Damn. Must have missed a step. I'll look into it.

I digress. Nurses. There are a great many who are perfectly fine, or perfectly wonderful, and I salute them. If they could have a word with their holier-than-thou counterparts, the veterinary world would greatly appreciate it. The rude ones, who pick apart authority and have been known to insist on us allowing them to do more skilled treatments at home themselves. You can imagine my secret thrill when one found out she wasn't as good as she thought she was at giving her pet fluids at home and admitted defeat.

While I'm curious about the comparisons in your human side of things when I go to my own doctor appointments, I wouldn't dream of assuming I know better than you. Respect our own wisdom and experience. Ain't rocket surgery.

The Less-Than-Shrewd

Not everyone is gifted with the same level of intelligence. That's a good thing, I suppose, so we're a diverse population of varying abilities, interests, and skill levels. I don't hold it against people who are, as the great Shakespeare would put it, "light of brain."

Some may take extra time to give discharge instructions, but I'll take that over an intelligent asshole any day of the week. My favorite is a client who, after you've spent time with thorough detail of the whole concept of the patient's diagnosis, the treatment options, the personally-tailored variables of their own life, and the final plan of execution, will then look at you with the blankness of a goldfish and say, "Ok, let's recap." So, you start all over. One time, it was just a recommendation to cut back on food portions for the dog. Seems pretty simple to say, "Feed a half-cup per day for Skittles," or, "Skittles needs a half-cup per day, but you can break that up into two feedings. Give a quarter-cup in the morning, and another quarter in the evening."

Easy, right? Not so. That turned into a twenty-minute discussion, because Skittles apparently doesn't have just one food bowl. Owner liked to have bowls to graze from on multiple floors of the home. Weird, I thought, when Skittles has no other companion dogs to compete against, but, ok? Still. No problem, right? "So, it's not too important where you put it, as long as Skittles has access. Let's still just make the *total* amount of food a quarter of a cup in the morning, between however many bowls, and ..." And it was still a difficult concept. She needed to know exactly how much to put in the bowl on the main floor, versus the upstairs, and what if she wanted to add one to the laundry room, or give a noontime treat, and, and, and.

Meanwhile, I mentally reviewed my breathing techniques. *At least she's not an asshole. At least she's not an asshole. At least she's not ...*

Some are blatantly, almost willingly ignorant, and that becomes even more frustrating.

Like the client I discharged from a routine preventive care appointment. I thought we'd looked the corgi-mix over pretty well, but hey, we're human and we sometimes miss things. The dog rolled over on the lobby scale for a belly rub when the owner suddenly noticed the spot, which they brought to my attention. I looked at it, and thought, *crap! We'll have to get them back in the exam room and have the vet take another look.*

"I'm so sorry we missed that. With a lesion like this, I'm concerned it might be some kind of ringworm. See how it's red and inflamed? Crusty along the edge of the circle? We can take Snickers back in and—"

"Ringworm? No, that's not ringworm."

"Well, I can't guarantee without doing some diagnostics on her, like taking a fungal culture. We could also rule out a bacterial inf—"

"You must have scratched her."

"I … scratched her? No, that's not a scrape, Sir, that's a lesion that—"

"No, you scratched Snickers with your watch when you carried her."

I pettily wanted to point out the face of my watch was a small *rectangle* and not even a typical round one to match the trademark-ringworm lesion on their dog's abdomen. *Ring*-worm! Round! Not rectangular. Even if it was the correct shape, why would it have left something more closely resembling a burn-mark, rather than a more linear scrape-mark? That's not how scratches work.

I ended up having to let that one go. You can't reason with some people. Made the ridiculous SOAP note addendum on the file that the owners dismissed my offer for a second diagnostic look, feeling the staff member's watch had accidentally scratched the dog during handling.

Never saw that one again, but I often wonder how long it took for the ringworm to spread and for that owner to move beyond the denial stage.

Speaking of. Flea-nial. Yes, you read that right. This is a widespread phenomenon, not a unique one. Folks in vehement denial that their sweet Rocky could possess fleas. *No, see, Rocky doesn't ever go outside*. Or, the infamous, *We live in a gated community, there's no way Rocky could have fleas*. A comparable scenario is intestinal worms. Clients frequently tell me they don't need that fecal test. *I already looked at Ellie's poo and didn't see any worms*. Followed by skepticism on their face when I explain that we usually detect parasites under the microscope, and can't rely on the naked eye. We don't normally wish life-suckers on any patients—ectoparasite or endoparasite. For the nonbelievers, though? We get a little smug when Rocky's flea comb comes up riddled with flea dirt and the incriminating little jumping beans. Or when Ellie's fecal test features those parasitic eggs winking back at us through the lens.

Another I couldn't convince was a sweet old lady who thought her dog needed his shoulders ice-packed after rawhide chewing sessions. She observed his flexed shoulder blades as he worked at the treat and assumed they must be sore. At least that wasn't going to hurt the dog, if he tolerated the ice. Wasn't worth the argument.

To contrast? The case brought in by a teenage guy, at his mother's insistence. The mother noticed when she dog-sat for her son, the canine guzzled down bowls of water like it was going out of style. She was perplexed, as Roxie was a young dog that seemed an unlikely candidate for diabetes or some other ailment. Still, she wanted to be sure, so she urged him to bring Roxie to the vet.

I started gathering my patient history in the exam room.

"So, your mom feels like she has to constantly refill Roxie's water bowl. How often do you notice you need to do it when she's home with you?"

"I don't know. I don't really do it that often. I guess I give her water every few days."

"Oh ... then, she still had water left in the bowl after a few days?"

Teenager shook his head. "No, I mean, she finishes it when I give it to her. And then I just wait a few days."

"You don't refill it ? … Immediately?"

"No? I give Roxie water a couple times a week."

After a little further clarification to be sure I wasn't insane, I thought I'd settled on the solution. Motherfucking kid wasn't giving his dog water; only a few scattered times in the space of a week. No wonder Roxie went on a polydipsic bender every time Mom dog-sat. I wanted to shake Teenager by the shoulders and ask him how often he felt thirsty? If he permitted himself a glass of water? But that's frowned upon from a professional, so I had to settle for the lecture of how it's important to give your pet access to fresh water *all the damn time, every single day*, while also trying not to sound like a condescending ass about it. (No mean feat.)

Boom. Healed.

What next? Ah, ignorance.

Ladies, if you're the primary caregiver for the pet, for the love of fuck, please stop sending your guy to the vet appointment in your stead. Unless you've given him a specific written list. He doesn't know anything, and when we get limited history or poor understanding of what you're wanting, it's not fair that *we* get blamed when something gets missed. ("Ma'am, he *declined* the heartworm test, and never mentioned wanting a refill on heartworm prevention …")

Oh, fuck off with any complaint of sexism. After the 93rd phone call from an irritated wife, I can gripe. Men are perfectly capable of being fantastic owners, but more often, they're just sent on the errand.

To tie this chapter up? Lunacy can be a matter of opinion.

I take little issue with pursuit of holistic methods of preventive care, when it doesn't ignore proven protection of modern medicine. I don't think it has to be an all-or-nothing approach. There's a benefit that would be stupid to ignore, that one should take care of their whole body, mind, and spirit, and not only a symptom in isolation. I can get on board with that. You won't hear me argue against the fact that the earth provides natural ingredients meant to keep us healthier and well-balanced. But I'll also argue there are times to admit the big guns are needed; that vaccines really work, that there's an anatomical ailment only surgical intervention can fix, or that you've got a raging infection requiring modern antibiotics.

We once had a nice gentleman present with his cat for urinary troubles. Common complaint. We ran the urinalysis to find a bad infection, as well as crystals that hinted at urolithiasis. We confirmed with a quick X-ray. Stones in the bladder. Thankfully kitty wasn't blocked yet. Still time to treat with an antibiotic and get her on the right diet to try to dissolve those stones. If things went well, the owner could avoid the expensive surgery and treat the cat conservatively. He nodded in understanding, perfectly agreeable to the recommendations.

In the middle of explaining how to administer the antibiotic, the man's wife swooped into the clinic. He must have called or texted her an update of what we'd found. She was less than agreeable.

Not rude about it, I'll grant her. But she gave us the placating, insincere smile of someone who might as well have said, "Bless your hearts." Like we'd guaranteed we could treat her pet with unicorn tears and phlegm from Nessie. Husband didn't argue with her. He went along, which told us he was probably used to having to keep the peace by being the submissive one. At least in this regard.

She grabbed the cat in its carrier, declined all treatment, paid for the exam and diagnostics only, and that was that.

Kitty was going to receive treatment via her own beliefs in holistic routes. None of our wild Western medicine, thank you very much. We were a little blindsided by the 180 the appointment had taken. We put the food and medicine back on the shelf and documented what happened.

As one of my tech school teachers once said, "Well. She made a choice. It's not the choice I would have made, but she made a choice." I've re-used that line many times. The polite response to 'Bless Your Heart,' and I appreciate it so much.

I wish I could be one of those people who takes the higher road to be glad of the ultimate good. The patient got taken care of, in this instance. Alas. You can't begin to imagine my smug satisfaction a month later when they returned. Asking for those antibiotics and the prescription food. Kitty hadn't improved with the holistic route. Weird. It's almost like we sometimes know what we're talking about.

Patients: I'm Abscessed

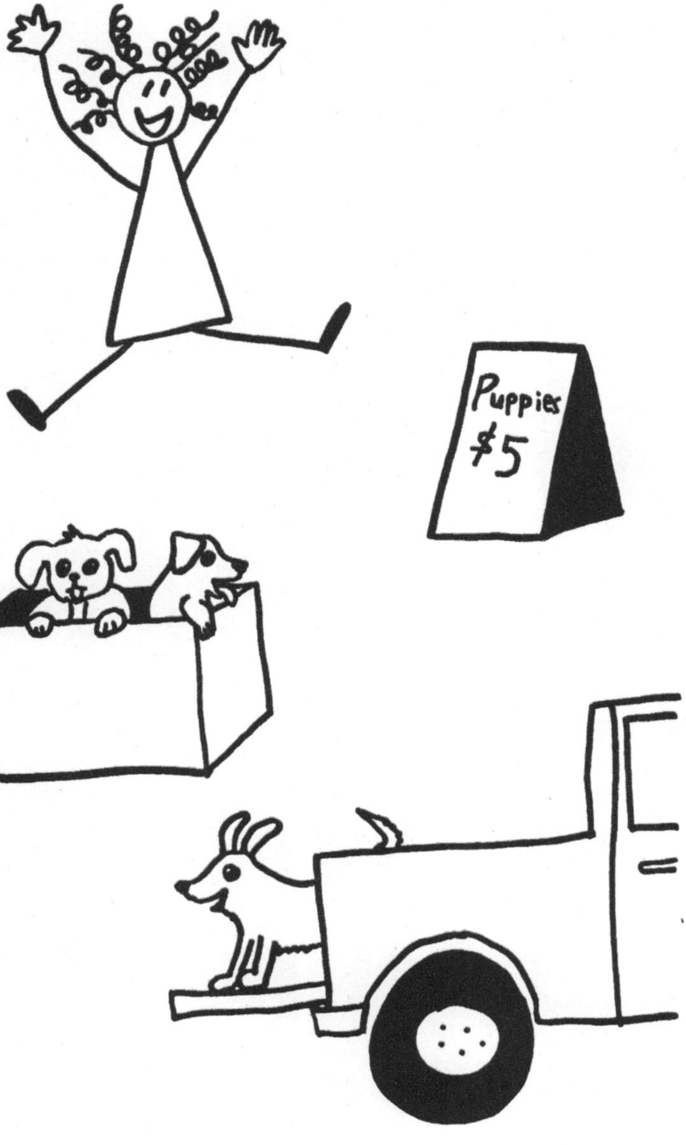

Embarrassing Emergencies

"How embarrassing to be human."
—Kurt Vonnegut

If you find yourself in the position of having what you deem to be an embarrassing emergency with your pet, do us the courtesy of being honest anyway.

My favorite honesty-award clients owned a golden retriever prone to ear infections. That's not an emergency, but when most people tend to lie or exaggerate to make themselves look like better owners, it was refreshing when they were so upfront about their dog's chronic issue. "Hey. The kids have had the flu and the house is a mess. So we've completely slacked on treating Tillie's ears and now they're awful again."

Hey. Thank you. Seriously. For acknowledging your humanity. Most clients would have lied to my face and sworn they were diligently administering meds, even though I can see (and smell) the neglected ears in front of me. Not them. Now we can move forward and address Tillie's ears today.

If your dog got into your stash of pot, we're more concerned with saving its life than we are about turning you in for possession. Seriously. Just tell us. We don't care about your extracurricular activity. We want the fast answer so we can jump into the correct medical procedures.

Though, maybe it was the side effect of paranoia that comes with being stoned that made those kids afraid to tell us, when they knew perfectly well what was wrong with their Chihuahua. Either way, at least they owned up to it, eventually. The distinctive lingering scent was certainly a clue for our veterinarian on call.

As for me, I'll admit, though the owners were currently in a panic, it was the calmest emergency patient I've ever encountered. As a fellow staff member and I were rushing to get an IV into the dog's front leg, it was hard not to laugh at the chill expression on his face. No cares in the world and not bothered a bit by the needles being jabbed in the vein for treatment. Just heavy lids and a dazed, glassy-eyed expression, characteristic of a pleasant marijuana high. A definite stark contrast from a typical Chihuahua disposition inside a clinic.

If dogs could talk, I expect he might have said something like, "Look how loud the colors are, man."

He lived, by the way. While marijuana is toxic to dogs and can cause alarming symptoms, most will come through it with therapeutic intervention. CBD products are an increasing fad on the market, even for dogs for various ailments, but please don't confuse it with your own human-grade THC shit. Keep your puppers out of that.

Know what else embarrasses people? Sex.

No, I'm not going there. But your pets may get into your personal items in that arena, if given the chance. Veterinarians have taken any number of strange items out of pets in a foreign body exploratory. One of my personal favorite stories occurred at a clinic shortly before I worked there. The lady reportedly showed up with her big dog. Knew exactly what it had eaten. Didn't want to talk about it. More or less just dropped the dog off, signed the consent forms, and said, "Fix it."

Too mortified to discuss the details surrounding the impressive wads of used condoms pulled out of the dog's stomach. Did the vet team have questions? Definitely. But they went unanswered, and in my opinion, it's better left an intriguing mystery.

Dogs love intimate items. Other favorites to eat include dirty underwear, dirty socks, used tampons and pads, and snotty tissues. All of these have been items required to be removed from GI tracts. My own male dog is guilty of finding my personal belongings to be a delicacy. I try to be careful, but it's hard even for me to keep him out of my laundry pile sometimes. Thankfully he's been able to pass everything he's eaten so far. I went out of town last week and dropped him off to board for a few days. My office manager later texted me a picture of the mess he'd made outside with the caption, "What the heck did your dog eat?"

Unfortunately, I recognized the distorted material among the muck.

"Ugh. Probably my jeans. Or my underwear. Do you want him? Good thing he's cute because he's fucking gross."

"No," she replied. "I already have a panty eating dog and I don't need another. Haha."

Lucky us. But we do try to tactfully warn some of our clientele of this behavior from their furred companions. Keep your personal equipment personal.

I've been asked an embarrassing number of times by owners calling in urgently after the rendezvous—

"So, is there any, like, Plan-B for dogs?"

That is one of those moments where we have to bite our tongues not to laugh at you. No. No, there is no animal equivalent of the morning-after pill for your horn-dogs. But hey, there's this great concept called spaying and neutering your pets! We recommend it!

The final notable emergency I'll mention was less of a private affair. More of a "How the fuck did that actually happen?" situation.

Cat in a dryer.

It seems like one of those implausible things from a sitcom, but it did happen. We got the harried phone call, and minutes later, the car came screeching into the parking lot. Somehow the kids closed the cat into the clothes dryer. Didn't think to check it for pets before turning it on. I'm assuming hysterical screeching eventually tipped them off to the problem.

In any case, Dryer Cat was the most frantic I've ever seen. Unceremoniously dumped onto the exam table, he sprawled his legs out like a flying squirrel mid-glide. The surface of the table must have felt cool to the poor hyperthermic feline, and he was desperate for any relief. I have to give the patient props for not clawing my face off in his panic. Under the circumstances, he was still a nice kitty, even as I rushed him to our bathtub and to cool him off under the water. Cat gradually calmed down, soothed by the relieving temperature, and was still cooperative as we monitored him over the next few hours.

Curiosity almost killed the … never mind, I can't do it.

Parvo-Land

"Canine parvovirus is a highly contagious virus that commonly causes GI disease in young, unvaccinated dogs. Presenting signs include anorexia, lethargy, vomiting, and diarrhea, which is often hemorrhagic. Diagnosis is typically based on history, physical examination findings, and fecal antigen testing. Treatment is largely supportive on an inpatient or outpatient basis because specific therapies are not available."
—Merck Veterinary Manual
(Alex Gallagher, DVM, MS, DACVIM-SAIM)

When I was in tech school, if any of the students were sick but still well enough to attend lecture, they were expected to isolate themselves out in "Parvo-Land." Not as magical as it sounds. It was just the unused half of the classroom, filled with empty tables.

These were pre-Pandemic days, for any young reader wondering why they didn't attend online. But as good VT students, caring about the welfare of our fellow comrades, we placed ourselves there when necessary. Our own self-appointed honor system. Schools are petri dishes during sick season. Illnesses abound. Hard to avoid transmitting our crud back and forth in close quarters between classrooms, labs, and locker bays. The isolation of Parvo-Land did help.

Parvovirus is not zoonotic. Meaning, it doesn't cross species. Humans can't get it from their pet canines. Still, the analogy helped to illustrate the contagion concept.

A dog's chances with parvo are about 50/50, my employing veterinarian likes to tell his clients. I couldn't say if that ratio is the most correct according to current scientific research, but it's probably close enough. It gives the clients realistic expectations when they get the unfortunate diagnosis.

There's no cure for parvovirus.* Only prevention, with the proper protocol of vaccines. Which is why we so staunchly recommend getting your puppy vaccinated, and from an ethical and trusted source, such as a veterinary clinic. Not your damn breeder. Not your local farm-supply store down the road.

All one can do is treat for the symptoms when a puppy or young dog—the most likely to be affected by it—comes down with the deadly disease. Parvovirus attacks the gastrointestinal tract, which causes the signature bloody diarrhea that owners tend to notice, sometimes with a mucoid appearance. There's a distinct smell any veteran veterinary staff member will detect and discern from your run-of-the-mill dietary indiscretion diarrhea. They'll tell you. "Smells like parvo." Owners will also see their precious pooch has suddenly become rather lethargic. Given the ability to take the dog's temperature, it would likely read at a fever level. Probably vomiting, too, if they've managed to eat anything in the first place.

It's a virus shed through feces of infected or carrier dogs, and it's highly contagious. I can't stress that contagion part enough. Hardy, easily transmissible, difficult to kill. Great combination, right? Good for the virus, I guess.

If you've walked through my house on any given Tuesday,

you'll notice I'm not the world's best housekeeper. I mean, respectable enough to be livable, but I'm not a germaphobe, nor a clean freak. When parvo or even suspected-parvo has set foot in my clinic, though, I become a different person. I'm the Sanitation Taskmaster. It's how I was taught. When I started at my small-town clinic, I noted immediately the blasé attitude about it. I upgraded the parvo protocol damn quick.

Any assistants trained by me know I want every imaginable surface drowning in virucidal-rate disinfectant. From the door handle that owner touched to get into the building, the floors of lobby and exam room, the front desk, the bathroom if the client even thought about using it, the pen they used to sign their paperwork—or better yet, just throw it away, the exam table that had better damn be saturated a minimum of three times, exam walls, exam chairs, exam instruments, foot-bath for anyone's tennis shoes who came near it, scrubs removed and replaced … I mean it. I want the clinic to smell like a swimming pool. If the odor of bleach doesn't make you say, "Oh my God," and cover your facial orifices, it's not good enough.

Yes, I do allow and expect the assistants to run outside for breaths of fresh air during the disinfection process. (I'm suffering through it, too.) But I'll never go to bed worried that I might have aided in the transmission of parvovirus to any vulnerable patient.

I've seen it enough times, I've long ago lost track of how many cases I've had in my career. Most follow similar patterns, though. Similar histories. A few notables among them. One of my very first ones, as a naïve veterinary assistant in the bigger city clinic, has irreverently become the butt of jokes between my husband and me.

If the reader is concerned, Husband doesn't get to know identities of clients or information about patients that might give anything away. HIPAA doesn't apply to animals, but there's still a sense of respect for client privacy. So, he may hear general details of interesting cases, as most medical professionals can probably attest to their significant others. But no more.

In this early case of my veterinary career, the client presented with their young pitbull-mix pup. A week or two before, according to the case notes I read, Puppy had tested positive for parvovirus. The veterinarian on the case was eager for me to get as detailed a history as I could first, before she came into the exam room. Apparently the young couple stood out in her memory, too. She was shocked the dog was still alive.

Like it or not, I've been doing this long enough to notice the patterns in parvo cases. Unfortunately, that pattern is that such cases come from poorly-educated or low-income clients. They are either too ignorant to make vaccination a priority, don't understand vaccine booster scheduling, simply can't afford it, or outright don't think it's important. Some of them blow more money than they should on the purchase of the animal, but don't factor healthcare in the budget. Some clients are just unlucky, too, and they have their space. But as kindly as I can say it, this couple fell into the first category.

My task was to get a clear picture of case updates and then present all pertinent information to the doctor. I tried to ask open-ended questions first. Followed up on any details they gave me, asking for more specifics. That's typical. This couple didn't care to talk much. I was pulling teeth to get answers from them. Had they pushed fluids since last time? Had they given the recommended antibiotics for potential secondary infection? How was the puppy acting? Past SOAP notes seemed to indicate they had declined most treatments, so what had they done? I tried to discover this via nonjudgmental query. Eventually, and with great hesitation, the probably nineteen or early-twenty-something young man admitted they'd been doing what they could to feed Puppy.

I pried further. "Ok, great. What have you been feeding?"

And eventually it came out. Not just feeding, but 'shotgun-feeding' the pup a mixture of puréed hot dogs, baby food, and milk. I tried not to show my shock as I wrote the vile recipe down on my note sheet for the doctor.

"And how long did you feed him that for? When did you stop?"

"... When he was done with the parvo," he said. Uncertain of the terminology, but he gave it a stab.

For as disgusting as it sounds, the food may have done the little guy some good. It was nourishment. Something to fuel the little body fighting for its life. The attending veterinarian, with her extremely high standards of care for medicine, was of course horrified at this unorthodox approach. She was one who struggled to ever compromise those gold standards. I'm sure it kept her awake at night. Nonetheless, their dog was alive and fit enough to receive a vaccine.

They got lucky. They came out on the good side of that 50/50 chance. I don't think they discovered the cure, but my husband and I have joked ever since about patenting that million-dollar idea. "Parvo-Cür," I think I'd call it. Keep it simple. I even did a silly sketch of what the product packaging would look like. A slick little tub featuring a cartoonish dog face, with its listed ingredients on the side panel. Hot dog purée +

Baby food + Milk. Mix it all up to create liquid parvovirus-curing miracle. Directions would indicate frequency and how many milliliters to shotgun feed your dog, by weight.

I had another young couple at the same clinic who were livid their dog had gotten sick. One of those thinking vet med was all a scam. That whole camp. They too, were lucky. Their dog had gotten a first distemper-parvo booster just before he had gotten sick. Little Norman probably already had the virus at that first appointment but wasn't symptomatic yet. After the puppy pulled through and they'd eventually come back to get their next booster, it took significant angry discussion, with the veterinarian sternly insisting they verbally state that they understood that we, the vet team, were not *giving* Norman parvo by administering the next vaccination. They repeated they understood, with great venom in their tones. Vet gave the injection, and they couldn't leave fast enough. They must have felt cheated in some way. Lied to. I couldn't speak to all the details of their case now, but I could say with some confidence that dog probably never received another vaccination again, due to their skepticism.

Where did public school biology fail so many? That's not a question I'm remotely equipped to answer, and educators will probably tell me with varying degrees of offense taken I'm not even asking the right question. It's just what I see in my narrow little pocket of the world. Maybe I hit the jackpot of biology teachers who knew how to expound on the miracles vaccines do for healthcare. I was lucky.

With those 50/50 odds, obviously I've seen the unlucky ones, too. And it's hard to predict.

I've learned not to forecast with any confidence to those owners who want me to have a crystal ball. Will their dog survive it, or should they cut their losses now? How much money will this cost them? Can they afford hospitalization and fluids? More often than not, we tell clients to take the dog home and push Pedialyte. Gatorade. Broth. Whatever they can. (Not Parvo-Cür.) Hospitalized fluids guarantee nothing, with that diagnosis. Is it the gold standard? Nah. Remember though, I'm usually trying to help someone who can barely afford the office exam fee, let alone the expensive test to confirm it's parvo-positive. I tell those owners, the pattern is that symptoms are usually apparent for a duration of about five days, at which point they desperately check the calendar, trying to count how many days back it first started. If puppy can get through those five days, that's what we hope for. We've seen puppies come in with mild symptoms, still acting playful or having a tolerable appetite, that were dead by the end of the day. Conversely, we've seen dogs come in like they're on death's door, and they turn around. So, we don't predict. We just wait and see for those full five days.

I try to stress the importance of getting those proper vaccine boosters—minimum of three sets of boosters (sometimes four, depending on breed, doctor-discretion, et cetera), each three weeks apart. Preferably starting at six weeks of age, or as close as possible afterwards. Not *before* six weeks of age. I'm talking to you, breeders.

Breeders tout all kinds of medical knowledge. I see breeder puppies every week in practice, have been in this field for at least a decade by now, and can still count on one hand the number of times I've looked over their information packets for their buyers and said, "Huh. Here's a breeder that knows what they're talking about."

Remember that, if you insist on having your pure-bred ball of joy—get the dog if you must but get the medical recommendations from the ones who actually have the degrees to back up their claims.

And to those owners who went the cheap route from their farm supply store? There's likely no stock-boy there who can properly educate you on how the life-saving vaccine should be administered. What complications to watch for. Or even that you're supposed to give multiple boosters on a set schedule, not just one. Hell, can you trust the part-time stocker even knew how to handle the vaccine shipment correctly? Stored at proper temperature? Did he advise you to do the same, or did you leave it on the passenger car seat while you ran other errands on the way home?

You don't know how hard it is not to be bitter when those owners call, in disbelief their dog got sick from something they vaccinated them for. Hell, it's tempting to tell you to fuck off and call the farm store where you got it. Ask them why your dog is sick. Yes, I've seen those puppies die. Numerous times. That's why it makes me so angry.

That's why when I receive vaccine records that came from a breeder, I'm checking their schedule closely. Or if you told me you or your cousin did your own vaccines and have stickers to "prove" it on an index card? Seriously? Just look at it. Does that look like an official medical record to you? Would you trust it? I know you're only in my clinic because you need to get the rabies vaccine for your legal requirement, but I'm still doing all I can to push my recommendation that you get another distemper-parvo booster from us. For good measure. To lessen your dog's chances of facing a fatal result. It's not a money grab. It's because I'm burnt out seeing unlucky cases.

The next biggest point I've learned the hard way? Stressing to those unlucky owners to *not* go out and get themselves another puppy after theirs just died. Fuck's sake.

You wish something like that would be common sense, when you've given the lecture on how contagious the virus is. What deep levels of cleaning and disinfection are required to decontaminate an environment. How unsafe and idiotic it would be, to bring another young, immune-compromised, unvaccinated dog into the same home where you just lost the other? And yet, I've had to field those conversations, when the owners are shocked to discover their second puppy has also gotten sick! You just want to scream and throttle them, but that's apparently unprofessional. I almost yelled at a dad who tried to blame his young son for the second puppy's repeat diagnosis. It was his fault, surely, for not taking out the trash, he said.

Seriously?

Fuck that. I made sure to say it wasn't the kid's fault. I weep for the home life that boy must have. But for my own failing? To be more thorough in my client education, going forward. Don't assume common sense is in place. Ever. Hell, I once had a guy tell me, after his pitbull fell out of the back of his pick-up and broke his leg (femoral head cracked, the radiograph showed, days after the fact), he'd been trying to help doggo get better by feeding chicken noodle soup. I don't mean to slight the powers of chicken noodle soup, but call me crazy —I think this wasn't its place. Certainly wasn't the answer I expected when I asked the owner if he'd been giving anything in the days since the accident, for pain. I hate to use the Lord's name in vain, but it's becoming a more regular occurrence for me.

Common sense, I miss thee.

Back to parvovirus. A shitty viral disease. One day, someone smarter than me will invent a Parvo-Cür that's legit. I hope so. At the time of this writing, there are promising new treatments in early marketing phases.* Likely to be released by the time this confessional rant is published. When they come out, I'm afraid they'll still be cost-prohibitive for the patients who need it. Its existence a moot point until it's affordable. We'll see. Until then, we have vaccines to prevent it. For the love of God, if you're thinking of owning a puppy, please do some research. Call your vet or your intended vet and ask them how much to budget for. If you can't afford it yet, save up first. Treatment is more costly than prevention.

—

*ADDENDUM:

Yep, there's an addendum. There was no parvo cure when I originally wrote this chapter. Lo and behold, the publishing process takes time and meanwhile, medical advances continued to develop. Within that window, parvo treatment was introduced to the market. Guess what? Some lucky ones may benefit, but the medication is expensive and cost-prohibitive for many.

For the Sake of Levity: Shrooms & the Cathouse

One tries to keep a professional tone when a client misuses medical or anatomical terminology. But let's be honest. It's the topic of many veterinary moments of levity.

Likely the most common flub is not knowing whether to use the term 'spay' or 'neuter' for their respective sex of pet. Which is why I *always* follow up the request with confirmation, to be sure they've mentioned the correct procedure.

"I need to get my dog, uh … spaded."

Spayed. They mean to say *spayed*. Not spaded.

"Ok, a spay appointment … And this is for a *female*, correct?"

"Ah, no, he's a boy …"

"Great. Let's check the schedule for a *neuter* appointment, then."

Some folks get annoyed by my follow-up inquiry, thinking I'm insulting their intelligence. When we hear the mistaken procedural terms as often as we do, well, forgive us for not trusting. I'm never mad about an initial mix-up from a client, so long as it's clear which surgery we're talking about for the final confirmation of the appointment.

And I'll never stop chuckling at "spaded." Respectfully behind their back, of course.

What else?

Bordetella bronchiseptica. Veterinary personnel will immediately know where I'm going with this one. Bordetella is the vaccine we give to dogs to prevent the most common strains of what's commonly known as 'kennel cough.' And most people prefer to call it that, in order to avoid the trickier word. "My dog needs that kennel cough shot."

We get it.

But you'll have to give us the grace that we're going to laugh when we hear the variations of the scientific name. It's even better when they're spoken with so much confidence.

"Does my dog really need to have that Portobello vaccine?"

Or,

"Yeah, I'm good with the Rabies and the Bordello shots today."

I mean, come on. The mushrooms are just funny. A plain portobello is actually safe for a dog to eat, so I hear. I've never fed mine any, but a vaccine against them seems wholly unnecessary. And if you know what a bordello is? There probably aren't enough vaccines to protect us all against that.

Charity Case 1: Eggs Benedict

"Give them love, because I believe that love can change, love can tame, and love can heal."
—Sangduen 'Lek' Chailert

Bleeding hearts are attracted to this field. That's just how it is. People who *love* animals to the point of making a career out of it are often the ones who can't resist something pitiful they can nurture until it's better. The warm fuzzies. We can't get enough of it.

One of the jokes in vet med is, sooner or later, everyone takes home a charity case. Some, more than others. When I started, I was a poor college kid, barely affording apartment rent and food. I still managed to be a pet owner by purchasing myself two sibling rabbits. One of them lived for over twelve years, the stubborn bastard. No, really. So much attitude in that delicate little guy. Though I'd had pets in my childhood, it seemed a responsibility to get a pet then, so I could relate to my clients. Otherwise, I was just some scam artist, right?

Well, a few years, some dogs, and a little more financial security later, I acquired my charity case. I'm admittedly proud to say he's the only one. Not that there haven't been other temptations. Maybe I should get out of the game before I become one of those professionals taking home multiples every year.

I had enough of a menagerie. At its peak, we owned six. I know that's nothing compared to some of you out there, but I lived in a small house and was selfish about my time. There were the aforementioned two rabbits—which, by the way, the sellers said were females: not the case. I didn't find out one was a male until the female was literally giving birth to six kits. When they were weaned, the kits found new homes. That was an education. But I digress.

Two rabbits. Three dogs. One snake.

We won't get into Miss Snakels, the moody corn snake. As for the dogs, we came by Java as the name for the mini rat terrier honestly. It fit her. As a puppy, she could vertically jump four times her height out of pure excitement, like an overcaffeinated pogo stick. Then, when Husband saw the picture of the old man Chihuahua with his obnoxiously bat-like ears from the shelter's photo, he immediately designated him Yogurt, before we even met the dog. Anyone who's a fan of Mel Brooks comedies will get that reference. We got those two shortly after our wedding, and they were our focus for a few years. Already, I noticed we'd inadvertently named both dogs after breakfast-related food items.

The charity case came later.

I went on a long lunch break one summer day, and when I returned, my veterinary assistant had an "Oh my God" story waiting for me. It was something to this effect.

Young man got dropped off at our clinic by a driver who was a stranger to him. Clearly, he was lacking his own transportation. He'd also apparently tried carrying his puppy to the *human* hospital in town first.

Take that in for a moment. Asking help for an animal at the human hospital? Can you imagine the look of ire from the receptionist? Endless phones ringing, processing insurance forms, patients desperate for appointments after arriving fifteen minutes late, and after getting coughed on by the latest virus-riddled swarm, in walks this furry would-be patient, that doesn't quite belong with the others in the waiting room. Anyway. Shocking nobody, they turned the guy and his canine away, after explaining what a veterinary clinic was. I'm not sure how far he walked, looking for help with his puppy, but eventually some Good Samaritan pulled over and gave him a lift to my place of employment.

The dog undoubtedly had a broken leg. His right front leg, to be precise, which he favored, putting no weight on it. Shaky history on how it happened. Still, pup was happy to dance around and beg for attention in his little kennel. He was an adorable fourteen-pound yellow lab-terrier-mix of some sort. Six or seven months of age, by our estimation. Apparently, the owner believed him to be a Great Dane. Let me reiterate, seven months old, and only fourteen pounds. For the non-Americans, 6.3 kilograms. Spoiler alert. He's not a damn Dane.

When someone struggles for transportation to our clinic and also makes the critical mistake of thinking the human hospital would fix the dog's leg, the veterinary clinic that receives it must make some judgment calls. Such as, besides being clueless, the kid probably has no money. We want to help any pet in need, but remember the part about having to run a business? We can't do everything for free, or else we can't afford to help the next patient …? Anyways. Yeah. That.

Before I'd even come back from my lunch break, doctor and VA realized that, and, pretty quickly, made their game plan. Radiographs were off the table, which obviously would have been nice. This was back in the day when we were still rocking films and such, before our digital replacement. Time-consuming and costly process. Kid couldn't even afford the office visit fee, so maybe we could waive that. Specialist care? Absolutely out of the question. Instead, out of the goodness of our hearts, we could sedate the poor pup and use a wire frame cast around his leg, bandaging it in place. His youthful puppyhood was on his side.

Gold standard? Hell no. But remember in practice, it's an all-too-common occurrence that financial constraints put us in the position of making compromises with treatment plans.

The young man was gone before I ever came back from lunch break, so I had to rely on the account from the doctor and VA. I arrived in time for the treatment plan and helped them carry it out. That wire frame was so old-school, I've never seen it before or since. Imagine something similar to the shape of a clothes hanger, but thicker-gauged, around the injured leg. Then, a complicated weaving of bandage material through, in, out, up, and around, so the leg never touches the frame, but is kept suspended in the middle of it. That's what poor doggo had to contend with when he woke up from sedation. Not that he complained. Animals adapt pretty quickly, and he learned how to swing it widely out and around. A half-circle sweep with every step so he could keep walking and playing around the hindrance.

So that young man was gone, but eventually, his girlfriend showed up. Honestly, the whole thing just felt … off.

She was upfront about not being able to pay us yet but would work on it. We told her to return in two weeks for a bandage change. Presumably she'd at least be able to chip away at the initial bill by then. We were already trying to cut her immense slack.

Thankfully, she returned two weeks later. We were all excited to see that cute pup. He had these Maybelline eyes, like they were outlined with eyeliner. A sweet disposition. Thrilled to see you. Just a good lab-mix. (Not Dane.) What was there not to like? Except the female owner was still unable to pay. A single mom with her deadbeat boyfriend, it didn't take us long to realize. We weren't without sympathy. The boyfriend never showed up again, after the initial drop-in.

What could we do? We were already invested in the treatment, and we had to continue. We did the next bandage change. Dealt with a pressure sore and added extra padding. Sent her on her way with a firm request she pay *something* by the next visit. In the meantime, that dog stuck with me. As a kid, I used to see Coca-Cola Christmas commercials with the picture-perfect Christmas morning. A yellow lab or golden retriever with a red ribbon around their neck for excited kids to unwrap on the holiday morning. And for a few years in a row, I asked my parents for that puppy for Christmas. Complete with red ribbon.

I knew by the third visit I loved that dog. While I enjoy a good puppy cuddle, I don't fall in love with every dog easily.

By then, the veterinarian/practice owner was reasonably concerned we were never going to see a dime from this patient's case. While we'd done the minimum to see the puppy through it (even throwing a courtesy distemper-parvo shot in there, since doggo had no vaccination history), we'd still invested time, energy, and resources. The doctor quietly pulled the client aside to stress the importance of payment. We didn't want to have to send her account to collections. To ruin her credit. Could she even pay a little? Talk to the manager about a payment plan to chip away at the ever-growing bill? She had nothing. And, she added in complaint that time: it was the boyfriend's fault. After all, he was the one that kicked the dog in the first place, so shouldn't he be the one financially responsible?

And there it was.

Suddenly our concerns had more grounding. The boyfriend (who we never saw again) had allegedly kicked the dog. Now it was an abuse case.

As an aside, I was starting to get an inappropriate, but itchy feeling I needed this dog. My house, shared with my husband and other pets, was small. We didn't have a ton of room for more. Still, I couldn't shake it. There was something about that puppy.

Weeks later, the lady was due to come back for the last of bandage changes.

Once more, the doctor hit her hard with the real talk, trying to do her a favor. This time, while they discussed money again, she had a second option which wouldn't ruin her finances. Not by us, anyway. That was to relinquish the pet, due to her inability to pay. For those unaware, if a client relinquishes their animal, they are essentially giving up all legal ownership of it when they sign that dotted line. They are no longer asked to pay the medical bills regarding the animal, but neither are they allowed to follow up with the pet in any way. He's not theirs anymore. If the pet gets euthanized immediately, or heroic efforts with specialist care are made to help fix X-problem? Either way, the client is no longer entitled to information. I've only seen three cases of relinquished pets in my decade-long career. Yes, it's usually sad.

I couldn't be in the room for that discussion, between the owner and the vet. Ethically, morally, I knew it would be wrong of me. But I waited eagerly to find out what she said. Fingers crossed she would see sense. Hoping I could take him home, I'd already confessed to the office manager how much I loved the dog. He was perfect, even with his wonky leg. Only his given name was stupid and cliché (not telling you what it really was, but we'll go with Bruno). How I would rename him Eggs. Eggs Benedict. He would complete my 'Breakfast Club' trio of dogs. Yogurt, Java, and Eggs. How fucking cute would that be?

The owner refused to relinquish that day. She loved Bruno, she said. How could she give him up? He was such a good dog, and great with her kids. They loved him. Besides, she promised us she'd dumped the original POS boyfriend and was dating someone new. New Boyfriend was surely going to help her out with the bill. Come to the rescue. She'd be back tomorrow and would take care of it.

I understood her quandary. The tight spot she was in. I felt for her. Didn't change that I also went home feeling devastated. The dog deserved a home that could care for him. His current family? While I didn't doubt there was affection for Bruno since the abusive boyfriend left, I knew more than I wished about their situation. That young, single mother needed to focus her finances on more essential things. Not vet bills. Still, we couldn't force her to relinquish. I wondered what kind of new schmucky boyfriend (who could have only been on the scene for a few weeks, at most) was going to walk in and pay for a puppy that had nothing to do with him.

Well, turned out …

When I knew the client was back the next day, I found something to do in the back radiology room. Something to clean. Anything to *not* be in the lobby, seeing the dog I desperately wanted and couldn't professionally handle.

After a bit, the manager came back to find me in the radiology room. She was holding the damn dog with the absurdly happy tongue lolling out of his head, despite his beaten-up e-collar.

"Hey, look," she said. "It's Eggs."

I sighed. Clearly she didn't understand how much it bothered me to see him.

"You mean Bruno," I corrected. Not amused. Not impressed. Wishing desperately she'd take him away so I didn't have to see him.

"No," she said more firmly. "*Eggs.*"

I probably tilted my head at her sideways. Confused. Until she spelled it out for me.

The dog was being relinquished, after all. The poor lady was in tears, and I would never gloat over that. But New Boyfriend had come into the lobby, asking for clarification on the situation. And once he understood if paperwork was signed, financial responsibility disappeared, he said the magic words.

"Do it."

He had zero intention of paying for his new girlfriend's bills, and neither should he have had to. Let's be honest, she should never have expected it. It wasn't his dog, and certainly not his problem. Might have been a gallant gesture, should he have been financially comfortable enough to handle it. But I couldn't speak to that. She signed that dotted line on the form.

I couldn't say whether they were still together as a couple for long after that. But I can say I got my dog. That same day, he got sedated for his final bandage and cast removal, got his overdue neuter procedure done, and a full round of preventive care he'd been sorely lacking. Hell, the veterinarian even gave me that day's services on the house. A gift, for being the one to take ownership from then on. We covered some of the previous unpaid bills with the Good Samaritan fund.

Eggs Benedict holds a special place in my heart. We tease him about whether he's a Good Egg or a Bad Egg on any given day. And every other egg-related pun or nickname you can think of. He learned his place in the household, with Yogurt the Chihuahua in charge, until we lost Yogurt, less than six months later, due to cancer. So, timing-wise, Eggs worked out perfectly. Found his place as a companion for Java and us, in time to help ease the loss of our old man.

He's a goofball of a dog 98% of the time, and the one I always wanted as a little kid. I don't force him to wear a red ribbon, but he does have a red collar in tribute to my childhood wish. I told the VA—the one who first saw him that fateful summer day—that if I ever woke up and found Eggs to have transformed into a Great Dane overnight, he would then belong to her. She had more room on her country property than my small house in the suburbs. While she might have been glad to keep him because there's a strong chance he's the best damn dog in the world, he's still managed to avoid a Dane-sized growth spurt. A fully-fledged adult now, he's less than twenty-five pounds. At least, when we haven't overfed him for begging with those seductive Maybelline eyes.

—

Did you think you'd get out of this chapter, unscathed from a SOAPBOX moment? Ha, cute. Hopefully folks in vet med will help vouch for me on this. We hear often, and sometimes, a half-dozen times a week, when someone claims their dog acts such-and-such way, "Oh, it's because he's been abused."

For the love of fuck, please stop. Unless you know with near-or-absolute certainty your animal's prior home abused them, resist this excuse. I'm not saying it doesn't happen. Eggs came from a home where his ass-wipe owner probably kicked him hard enough to break his leg. Every once in awhile, he gets a little stressed out if Husband and I are goofing around in the kitchen (Husband is a martial arts fan) and Eggs perceives it as a real fight. That type of thing. Then, he grumbles a bit or whines harder. He's submissive about being petted (still desperately wants to be petted. Please!). But that's about the extent of his 'abused' personality.

We hear frequent variations of, "My dog doesn't like men, and we think they were abused by a man once, so …" before they request their vet *not* be a man, if possible. If that many men were out there abusing dogs, I think half the male population in my town alone must wake up every morning, look at their alarm clock and think, "Oh, shit, my deadline! Better get to punching dogs!" You know. Quotas to meet.

What's really lacking? In my opinion, training, behavior, and breed awareness.

I implore you. Research dog training and behavior, if you haven't. Even if you think you do know how, refresh again. Just a few tips, even for basic commands. And especially to understand your own behavior, from the animal's perception. Know the proper leash or harnessing for your animal, too. If you've got your retractable leash ready, you can fix that by throwing it in the trash and getting a proper one. Especially if your pet is larger than fifteen pounds. I'm not going to spend time explaining why those mechanisms are the devil. They are. It's not up for debate.

And hopefully before, but even if it's after, do some damn research about your dog's breed. People will get up in arms about my saying this, and I'll touch more on my breedist opinions later, but let go of your ego and do it. If you didn't pay attention in Principles of Biology, both nature and nurture play a role in the outcome of a living organism. It's important to understand why your animal operates the way they do. What drives them. What their breed-specific needs are. Food, healthcare, energy, body composition and anatomy, intelligence, all of it. If you acquired a working dog, like a shepherd breed, and are just keeping them in your small apartment with the occasional walk around the block? You're going to have a bad time, and so is your pet. It's not fair to them. It's unrealistic for you to keep up with their energy needs. You're about to have a badly-behaved creature that's destructive and an anxious mess, because they don't have the proper environment to fulfill their functional needs. Too often, we see the results of a behavioral outburst that went too far, a violent clash, or just the sad situation of rehoming due to poor planning.

When people tell us their pooch must have been abused before, it's usually pretty plain to us they're just not well-socialized. Or not well-trained. Submissive behaviors such as cowering and shaking are common. Some breeds are more apt to take on an assertive stance. Or an aggressive posture. Some of those reactions may be out of fear, sure. It's probably because they're in an unfamiliar situation or don't trust the new person.

While I won't imply that there are no training challenges, I ask that the majority of you stop hiding behind the abuse-trope. Be smarter about training and breed requirements ahead of time, so that you don't have a heartbreaking situation later.

Charity Case 2: Winnie the Experiment

"No pessimist ever discovered the secret of the stars, or sailed to an uncharted land, or opened a new doorway for the human spirit."
—Helen Keller

I probably earn some kind of monstrous label for admitting I don't get the hype about corgis. I mean, I guess they're cute, with their buoyant butts and all.

From a veterinary perspective? They're popular farm dogs that can come with an attitude. You have to hope you get a nice one. And those stubby little legs just give me anxiety about having to draw blood, too. Vets will understand the venipuncture stress. I've been seeing one needing routine CBC checks every few weeks while undergoing chemotherapy. Sweet dog, I admit. But for a day I was going to be out for vacation, even the manager of my clinic asked me to write down the best anatomical location for the veterinarian to attempt while I was absent. Super medial access-point of the left cephalic vein is her best spot, by the way. Good luck finding the jugular in that thickly-furred, chubby neck.

But that's not even the corgi we're talking about.

We're talking about Winnie.

Winnie belonged to good, long-time clients who were straightforward, no-nonsense kind of people. Though, they would always balance themselves with kind generosity. They might run through a drive-thru and bring all staff back breakfast or lunch while you vaccinated their animals. Or a new seasonal knick-knack to replace the clinic's lobby décor that wasn't to the wife's taste. Some staff found them disconcerting. Too abrasive, sometimes. I wasn't immune to the irritation of their sass. The wife, especially, could get my goat if she wanted to. Like the time she didn't like the surgery drop-off time because it was earlier than she cared to be awake. Overall, I liked her for her strong opinions and tenacity for banter. I didn't have to sugarcoat anything when it came to their many pets. Just gave the medical opinion straight, and they'd return a straight answer.

"Yes, fix it," or, "Nope, not gonna bother with that. It is what it is."

Winnie the corgi must have been six or seven when I started seeing her frequently. She began having urinary issues and we did the typical protocols of treatment for urinary tract infections. Urinalyses and rounds of antibiotics. When symptoms kept recurring, radiographs to rule out bladder stones. Prescription diets and cranberry tablets. More antibiotics, again and again. Urine culture sent to our outside lab. At some point, she had a cystotomy performed by another clinic, when ours was unavailable to schedule it in a timely manner.

The end result was the bladder problems continued, even post-surgery.

Having an animal that has little to no control over their

bladder becomes maddening. The animal can't help it, of course, but I feel for owners going through it.

Winnie had to go frequently, as one with a UTI often does, and she often presented with varying degrees of hematuria—blood in the urine. Blood would stain the hair on her backside. This was no fault of the owners. They did everything they were asked. I had confidence in their compliance. Strict diets and all. Diligent about giving the medications. They weren't the type to allow a dog to get away with bad behavior or spitting out pills. Maybe that's one of the reasons I liked them.

They skipped a specialist, which may have shed light on things sooner, but I will never judge anyone that has to say "no" to that route. If I'm being straight, through most of my career, I would have struggled to afford taking my own animal to a specialist. And I work in the field. I'm still not paid well enough to think about it on my own, but my husband has a better-paying job, and I'm fortunate in that.

Back to our canine. Try as the owners might, Winnie waxed and waned. Even at her best, you couldn't say she fully improved.

After endless months of rechecking and more antibiotics and frustration, I didn't blame them for saying they'd had enough. The owners presented us with two potential proposals. Put Winnie down, or we could keep her and try to fix her ourselves.

I don't remember now how much debate went into it. However much there was, Winnie became one of the few pets I've seen relinquished. Signature on the dotted line and all.

Plenty of vet clinics have a clinic cat. Hell, we have more than I could want. But I bet there are far fewer boasting an office corgi. Winnie became ours. Often gated to the side lab room where she could still see people come into the lobby, or leashed behind the desk, most everybody loved the new greeter. She was cute, you had to admit. What most clients didn't see were the million potty pads in her area, spotted with persistent bloody urine. Besides that, the corgi wasn't terribly concerned with good aim. Our mop got a lot of use.

She became a pill about taking her pills. We learned to change the method of hiding them every week, before she figured it out. Keeping the integrity of a strict urinary diet wasn't having much effect anyways, so we allowed ourselves to use whatever treats we could to get her to take the medicine. Peanut butter and cheese were old news. We had to get more creative. Hot dog pieces, marshmallows, or even cheese puffs, if you could insert them gently enough into the crispy orange ball without it crumbling in half first.

Deceptive treats aside, no matter what therapies we tried, nothing worked for us, either.

Some months later still, things finally came to a head. Normally Winnie was bright and alert, besides what was probably uncomfortable urination. But then she went downhill fast in a matter of days. She suddenly became completely lethargic. Lost energy. Lost interest in food. Her eyes became filled with green discharge and she seemed to grow rapidly weaker. Once more, a decision needed to be made, and this time it was wholly ours. We either needed to end the poor girl's suffering, or we could do an exploratory surgery on her bladder. See what was there, after fruitless therapies and an already once-performed cystotomy.

We couldn't just let her die. It was obvious she was going to. We had to give her a chance. I wouldn't have been able to sleep at night if we hadn't tried. I may not be partial to corgis, but by then Winnie had lived at our clinic for months, and I loved her.

Point of fact, I didn't sleep well that Friday night. The plan was for the veterinarian and part-time VA to work their normal Saturday shift until noon, and then when the clinic was closed for business, we would perform the surgery. I volunteered to help on my day off.

I'm not one to get too nervous about a procedure, but I'm not usually so emotionally attached to the animal being operated on. My husband would tell you when we went out to breakfast that morning, my hands were shaking in anticipation. If we found nothing, or something dreadful, we would euthanize her, rather than waking her up.

I got to the clinic at ten 'til noon, and our doctor was already getting things rolling. I calculated our necessary drugs, shaved her, prepped the incision area, intubated her, and monitored her vitals under anesthesia. Then the doctor needed my help, too. Sometimes VTs just need to become an extra set of hands; to hold relevant vessels or organs out of the way, or hold tautly if the surgeon is trying to suture or manipulate something. I gloved up with sterile technique and left the machine controls to the VA. Winnie's bladder was located, and it was immediately apparent how unhealthy it looked. Reddened and scarred. Past surgery scar visible, too. The vet could tell as soon as he cut into it with his scalpel that the wall was thickened and inflamed. None of that was terribly surprising, given the patient's history.

What was surprising was that we found not stones, but a formed material of another kind in Winnie's bladder.

"What the hell is that?" all three of us verbalized. Whatever it was, it didn't belong.

It was light gray, almost the color of watery bird poop. Not exactly solid, either. The doctor picked at it with his gloved finger, and then with hemostats. A consistency almost like gunky toothpaste. Or what you might scrape out of your shower drain. It didn't come out in one fell swoop, but with continual plucking and flushing. As the doctor and I kept at it, the VA hurriedly started researching possibilities on her phone. It's scary that's the boat Winnie was in, but that's the truth of it. We didn't know what we had found. As we were finishing our task, she had not located any of the typically-available veterinary resources to identify the mystery-gunk, but instead, some convoluted scholarly research articles that may have shed some light.

One of them seemed to describe something similar to what we were seeing and had a few comparable case studies. We had to go with it as our guide. With that, we decided to consider the mystery gunk as some kind of bacterial plaque which had lined Winnie's bladder. Likely a *Corynebacterium* species, but we can only ever say that was our suspicion. The article also pointed us in the direction of a new antibiotic. One that had been on our shelf the whole time, but not the kind you typically reached for with bladder cases.

We got to wake Winnie up from surgery that day. And quickly, started her on the new antibiotic regimen.

She improved, at long last. Not only was she back to feeling better, but the problematic symptoms cleared up over the following weeks.

With a new ray of hope for her future, we had to consider her adoptable. Keeping an office-corgi forever is pretty unpractical. We didn't even have a chance to advertise her to a good home, though. The VA who helped research the probable *Corynebacterium* cause ended up taking Winnie home. Told you, all of us are guilty! That VA graduated from college and moved away to a new town, new home, and new career in a research-oriented field. She still sends us pictures of Winnie on her birthday.

Charity Case 3: Harper

"When you realize the value of all life, you dwell less on what is past and concentrate more on the preservation of the future."
—Dr. Dian Fossey

My stint with Harper was much shorter than the previous cases, but still impactful. I should probably start out by saying she wasn't relinquished, either. You might otherwise be concerned that's our clinic's Tuesday special.

She was a sweet boxer-mix. Might have even still had her full, natural tail, but my memory is vague on that point. What I do know is she belonged to a nice family. Considerate parents, well-behaved kids. Just good people.

Harper first presented to the clinic with GI symptoms. It eventually became a concern that she might be a foreign body patient. As in, she ate something she shouldn't have, and it wasn't passing. I imagine the human field sees their share of these, too, but veterinarians probably more so. Who can say? Somebody, but not me.

Harper's family struggled financially. When you don't have a lot of extra money lying around, you get concerned about going to a doctor. Or an animal doctor.

Harper's family were able to afford the exam, but they'd put it off for a few days first, hoping she'd get better, and it wouldn't be necessary. She didn't improve, so they bit the bullet for their beloved family pet. But it couldn't stop there, she needed more. Diagnostics to figure out what's wrong with your animal add up quickly. And when we found out an obstructive foreign body was what we were dealing with, the tough predicament started.

Foreign bodies can be fickle. More often, they are extremely urgent. Sometimes the item may not cause a blockage, per se, but can still be devastating to the intestinal tract. Like cats that play with string. Long, linear objects that, if swallowed, are dangerous, slicing tissue, or causing the intestines to bunch up.

If the foreign material *is* causing a blockage, what then? Having something stuck in your stomach or your gut that can't pass through is not something that can wait. The animal will usually struggle to eat anything else, if they even feel like trying. Attempts often result in vomiting. Neither are things passing effectively at the other end. Lethargy happens. Usually noticeable discomfort about their abdomen. And once again, a big blunt object, or something getting twisted in the intestine, will damage it.

Twelve hours, twenty-four hours, thirty-six hours can all make a difference.

If it's not obvious by now, Harper waited far longer than that.

The family were presented with the options. They knew they couldn't afford the surgery she needed to save her life. Neither were they ready to just select euthanasia, either. In their own way, they felt they had to try, too. And so, they did. Making whatever calls, rallying whatever troops they could for financial help. The unfortunate part? That still took time.

By the time they had secured funds and came back asking for the procedure, the boxer-mix had gone far beyond what a veterinary surgeon hopes for.

The veterinarian and I performed the surgery, nonetheless. While she was open on the table, it was plain some of her intestinal tract had become necrotic, meaning the tissue was dying. The telltale odor hits you in the face. If she was to have a chance, we wouldn't just be cutting into the intestinal tract to remove the blockage, we'd also be removing an entire section of extensively damaged intestine. The healthier ends are painstakingly sutured back together to re-form the tube shape, once the necrosis is cut out. This process is called an anastomosis. In truth, we discussed it during the procedure. What was Harper's prognosis, after this? Were we doing what was best for her?

At the time, we felt we were giving her a fair chance.

I won't delay the results longer. She didn't bounce back after surgery as much as we would have liked to see. The family was still so grateful. The mother made a crocheted basket with decorative dog bone-shaped handles on it. The kids helped her bake cookies, and they stuffed that little basket full, bringing it to us in thanks for our efforts. Meanwhile, Harper still acted rough. But we saw enough slight progress to eventually discharge her home, after a couple of days. Mostly in the hope she would feel better surrounded by her family, rather than in the clinic.

It didn't work. As well-intentioned as we'd tried to be in our choice during that surgery, we should have done the opposite and recommended putting the dog to sleep. Harper died horribly at home. In pain and bleeding, the owner told us. Not with blame. They were too kind for that.

In Greek, the word *euthanasia* means "good death" and I believe it is, in the right circumstances, a kindness the veterinary profession can offer to a patient.

I couldn't eat any of the remaining cookies after that. There was too much guilt for me. But I kept that crocheted basket in my surgery room. It's still there today. I can no longer change the devastating results of Harper's case, but the basket reminds me of that failure. Not for the sake of self-flagellation, but so I'll remember to do better for the next case. Sometimes harder decisions must be made, for the ultimate good of the patient. Kindness has to win out over sexy heroics.

Since Harper, it has happened again. Many other foreign body patients, saved. Rope toys, ballet shoes, a sewing needle with thread still attached, Mickey Mouse figurines, carpet fuzz, socks, and hygiene products have all been successfully retrieved. One did not come out of surgery, but I rest easier over it, knowing the damage we found during that patient's procedure called for that tougher decision. The kind decision.

You Are What You Eat

"My doctor told me I had to stop throwing intimate dinners for four unless there are three other people."
—Orson Welles

Food is the best medicine.

I never imagined I would talk about pet food as much as I have over the course of my career, but it's one of the most frequent topics of concern from owners. Are they feeding the right food? How much should they be feeding? How often should the pet be fed?

No, I'm not here to tell you there's a one-size-fits-all answer, because there isn't one. No panacea. No magical formula fulfills the needs of every patient.

I can tell you there's an epidemic of pet obesity, and that's the most common conversation surrounding nourishment that takes place. Has to be done somewhat delicately, though. As it would with a human patient (I imagine), folks are often sensitive to being told their pet is overweight. Pets don't feed themselves, so the obvious deduction is to place fault on the hand that does the feeding. "Looks like Dobby's finding his way to the food ok," my veterinarian usually remarks, when he enters the exam room. An attempt at humor to soften the blame.

For myself, I try to stick with the gentle nudge. "Well, Yoda's gained twelve pounds since last year," or the more goal-oriented, "Yoda's a little heavier than we'd like to see. A good weight for him would be closer to …"

Perception may be part of the issue. I think a lot of folks just don't see it. Instead, they're accustomed to the heavier pet as the norm. They don't know the markers to look for on their animal. A nice tummy tuck from the profile view. A waist, when viewing from above. Ribs should be palpable (but not visible) and not require you to press hard to feel them. We use body condition scoring charts to rate where they fall, in a number range assigning them somewhere from underweight, to ideal, to overweight. The scale is either out of five, or nine, with the lowest number being emaciation, and the highest as obesity. Mid-numbers are the model.

One time while occupied on a phone call on my back porch, I didn't notice I'd left the gate open. Suddenly I realized I hadn't seen my dogs in the last twenty minutes while I'd been chatting away with a friend. I hung up in a panic, starting out into my neighborhood and calling their names. The elderly Chihuahua was found immediately and easy to secure. He hadn't gone any further than sniffing the neighbor's flowers in the front yard. A good ol' Mama's boy, he was just happy to see me. The younger rat terrier was nowhere in sight. I walked up and down our street, calling for her. Eventually a neighbor several houses away noticed my distress and told me they'd found my pooch. Concerned she was skinny and had been going hungry, they'd quite efficiently found a can of dog food and fed her.

She was gone less than half an hour, by the way. Didn't starve in that time, I assure you. But it always struck me they saw my rat terrier as underfed. I'm sure she enjoyed her outing immensely with that unexpected treat, but for the record, by veterinary standards, she's an ideal body condition scorer.

There's a surplus of clients who don't like to admit how much their pets get to eat. They're hesitant to own up about feeding table scraps. If not that, how many treats a day the pet receives. If they free feed, rather than on a schedule. Or, the cup they use to dump food in the bowl is a Route 44 Sonic size, rather than any proper measuring cup.

On the contrary, some are oblivious. One of the best conversations between our vet and a client entailed her asking about his morbidly obese Min Pin's daily feeding habits.

"Oh, not that much at all!" he assured her. "In the morning, he gets his kibble. And then one of those Little Cesar's packets. Oh, and then a small bone whenever he potties. And then kibble at lunch. And then some canned food when I sit down to read the paper. Oh, and we do a 3:00 p.m. cheese bite as well, and then …"

He still didn't hear it, even as he addressed each treat. Baffled as to why we were concerned about the dog's muffin top.

Some general feeding tips for the stressed owner:

- Feed fewer treats, simply by breaking them into smaller pieces. You don't necessarily have to adjust the daily routine. Just give less of the treat. Pets don't make a fuss that they're only getting a fourth of a treat at a time. They only know it's a reward.
- Scheduled feeding times are better than free feeding, if weight loss is recommended.
- Use their own kibble as a treat, for food-motivated pets and especially training purposes. Whatever was allotted for the daily feeding regimen, take a small portion for

training time instead. Fewer unnecessary calories are consumed.
- Dry kibble is better for dental health. The mechanics of chewing causes friction of the harder food against the surface of the tooth, making it more difficult for dental calculus to adhere. Unless there's a medical reason to offer canned options, stick with dry.
- Multi-pet households often mean there's competition at the food station. Those pets are more likely to scarf down their bowl before the housemate gets it. Maybe they're well-matched against each other. Maybe there's a disparity between who's the dominant/food-aggressive one at the station, versus the submissive one who gets by on less sustenance. Single pets may take their time about their food because no one is lurking nearby to steal it.
- Use a fucking measuring cup. Seriously. Figure out the recommended amount for your pet and use that marked line as your guide. Your vet clinic probably has hundreds of freebie measuring cups from their prescription food suppliers. Ask for one.
- No table scraps. Or at least, extremely sparing. Being a pound overweight isn't terribly significant to a human, but that's substantial to a domestic animal.

You get what you pay for when it comes to food brands. The key point to remember is, while you could buy that mega-bag for cheap at Wally World, it's shit quality. You have to feed Mr. Frodo a lot more filler garbage to get to the caloric number he needs to sustain himself. On the flipside, when you buy the more expensive stuff, Mr. Frodo doesn't need nearly as much. More quality to those calories. In theory, you're not saving many pennies by buying the cheaper option, if you know how to feed correctly. Besides that, there's less output in your yard to clean up, when you feed the better shit.

What about the in-betweens? Sure. There are middle-of-the-road options that are fine on a budget. There are also extremely popular ones on the market that aren't necessarily high-quality food. Really, just average. But their marketing strategies are excellent. Drawing consumers in with attractive packaging and bold claims touting the supremacy of the ingredients. Meanwhile, they're often appealing to trends in human diets which make owners feel warm and fuzzy.

Beware those fad diets. I wouldn't dare lecture anyone on human nutrition, but don't expect what's good for you to be good for your pet. The grain-free trend is one of the worst offenses. Deny yourself all the grains you want, but there's plenty of evidence now coming out to show the catastrophic long-term effects it has on your pet. They require grains for heart health, and feeding the deleterious diet has been linked with canine dilated cardiomyopathy. Cats may develop hypertrophic cardiomyopathy. If that sounds like bad news, it is. Both can be fatal.

I'm not a fan of raw diets, either, if anyone's asking. There's a hell of a lot of options purchasable online or on the shelves for raw food. But a lot of it is unregulated by FDA standards, and as it would be a risk to humans, uncooked proteins can harbor unsafe bacteria that will cause illness to your pet. One of my vets has a Labrador we swear could eat anything and never die. GI tract never fazed by the outdated leftovers he's offered. Lucky him with his great genes, but he's in the minority. Alas, a good many of my patients might be offered even a different flavor of their regular food brand and suffer blowout diarrhea for the switch. Our household pets may be descendants of wild animals, but we're many generations removed from that now, and I can confidently say my miniature rat terrier doesn't closely resemble a wolf gnawing on its fresh kill. I don't eat raw hamburger, and neither will she.

"Well, I guess you and I are different people, then," one of my clients snarkily told the vet, when he asked her opinion of feeding raw burger meat to his Yorkie. Missing the irony that this was the very reason he was paying for the vet visit. Severe GI upset. Still wasn't ready to own up to his mistake.

Some attitudes we just can't fix.

We carry lines of veterinary prescription foods, and that means what it sounds like. We hope your pet doesn't require it, because when such food has to be prescribed for a medical condition, it's expensive. There are a handful of brand options, but the price hurts, regardless. Numerous variations of gastrointestinal foods, liver, kidney, thyroid, metabolic, weight management, and urinary diets are what you will find on your vet's shelf. Most of them are restrictive diets. Especially urinary health ones. Other outside foods, whether over-the-counter brands or table scraps, interfere with the medical purpose of scripted food. If you're paying the exorbitant prices because your pet needs it, don't let it all go to waste by offering nibbles on the side. Then we have problems that could have been avoided. Those clients end up coming back for a recurring problem when they deviate from the script, often because they found something at their grocery store marketing itself as being urinary-health-friendly. Friends, it's not prescription-grade, and it's not enough. That ended up costing those clients more money in the end.

We give medicines to pets everyday as preventatives and treatments for all manner of ailments. The stuff they put into their mouths daily to function greatly informs their overall health. Organs, skin and coat, dental hygiene, energy level, all of it. We get asked for brand recommendations all the time, and we're happy to give them. Apart from the prescription stuff on our own shelf, I promise we're not making a profit from the other suggestions. Sometimes folks are paranoid about that. I wish I could give them reason to be, but we get nothing out of it, other than a patient hopefully on the right track.

Feed your little buddies to the best of your ability. We want you to.

Bon(e) Appetit.

For the Sake of Levity: Tempering Expectations

Another of those silly vaccine mix-ups. I'd heard of this legendary misunderstanding before but presumed it to only be that. A legend. Surely no one actually assumed …?

And then one day it happened. It really happened.

The tremendously polite gentleman client presented with his brand-new pup, excited to get started. Over the course of discussion about how things had been going so far with puppy training and a review of what we planned to accomplish during the appointment, he was eager to request a particular vaccine.

"Oh, I want to make sure I get that distemper shot," he said. "Because he's been biting me a lot, and I'm hoping that'll make him nicer."

I sat there stunned for a few seconds, trying to collect myself for a response. Torn between wanting to applaud his willingness for the highly-important vaccine, but also to manage expectations about what a distemper vaccination is capable of achieving. It broke my heart a little bit to burst that bubble for him.

While distemper vaccinations, when correctly administered, help to prevent a terrible disease, I cannot claim they will do anything to eliminate your doggo's bad temperament. I could do nothing for the improvement of puppy's disposition that day, but I did protect him from fatal canine illness.

Love Hurts

"I have studied many philosophers and many cats. The wisdom of cats is infinitely superior."
—Hippolyte Taine

Sometimes in life, you have to make the call for the ultimate good of the situation, even though there will be collateral damage in the process. In veterinary medicine, we want to do what's best for the animal. Try, though, as we might to minimize stress, sometimes to accomplish vital treatment, it's hard on the patient.

As a quick aside, hey clients? While I appreciate any helpful warnings you can give us about ill behavior or concern ("Piddles will need a muzzle when you do her nails,") on the flipside, it's rude and demoralizing to make jokes or comments about how much your animal doesn't want to be there. Yeah, we already know. We're dedicating our time and energy to making it as smooth as possible because we care about your creatures. We know it's still scary for them. We can see them planting their feet and having to be dragged in the lobby. Tucked tails and anxious drooling. Hackles raised and shifty-eyed glances. You don't have to spell it out. I've literally had someone tell me, the second I walked in the exam room and barely got out the hello to the client I'd never met, "Oh, he hates you. He only likes me and Dr. A." No other introduction.

Fair warning, I guess, but damn. Fuck you, too.

Not everything is hateful when it comes to see us. We have jolly patients, too. Or at least, content ones. The ones we're excited to feed peanut butter and cheese treats.

One such patient was a longhaired fluffy orange kitty I'll call Sprout. We saw Sprout numerous times, starting with her kitten vaccine appointments. Friendly, lovable cat. Always did well. Nice clients.

Until the day I got a frantic call from Sprout's owner that she had eaten part of their Easter Lily around the holiday time. Deadly to a cat. Any part of a lily—stem, petal, leaf, pollen—can be dangerously toxic and cause kidney failure. Cat owners should steer clear of having them in their homes. It was an honest mistake, of course, and this particular owner was beside himself with worry. He rushed her in shortly after having discovered she'd eaten it. The attending doctor let me take the lead on administering the activated charcoal to sweet Sprout. Meant to act as a binding agent to the toxins going through her GI tract, so that it minimized organ damage and helped her to pass the offensive material more safely.

I went as gently as I could, but as our vet likes to tell people: "Cats live and die by their own rules."

Sprout started getting impatient with me mid-way through forcing the charcoal dilution down her throat. By the end of her dosage of it, she was furious. Then we had to try for fluid therapy, and we did as much as she would allow. After that? Poor Sprout. At her limit. I didn't blame her. Animals have little sense of correlation in this situation, of action and corresponding reaction. She had no idea why she was rushed to the vet and was having foul liquid syringe-fed to her, or being poked with needles. She just knew it was happening and didn't like the rude event one bit. It was agreed we should keep her for monitoring, so we set her up in our cat ward for the night.

The owner was a nervous person and very upset about the whole thing. Sobbed in his car in the parking lot before he left. He called numerous times throughout the rest of the workday to check in on her. To see if Sprout had calmed down, firstly, and then if there was any sign of illness yet apparent. It's hard to reassure an emotional person sometimes, but we tried to convince him Sprout was better left without us peeking in at her every five minutes and stressing her further. The sweet kitty was no longer there. At this point, Sprout had turned into one of those demonic felines you can only catch with gloves or a pole. Ready to unleash hell and bite or scratch anything that dared get close to her kennel. Hissing, spitting, yowling, all of it. All we could do then was monitor. Preferably through the window looking into the cat ward, instead of approaching her kennel.

I dreaded going into work the next morning to deal with the pissed-off Sprout, but found before I'd even arrived, the owner had come and gone before me. After a sleepless night, he'd been waiting for the first staff member to arrive. Gathered Sprout in the first minutes of the clinic opening and whisked her off to the nearest specialist and urgent care veterinary hospital over an hour away.

The reports from that hospital trickled in later. I believe they had to sedate her to be able to do much, but the eventual bloodwork showed values as being stable. She had minimal to no signs of the toxicity, and the doctors there told the client I'd already saved Sprout's life.

The solution to pollution is dilution, the old adage goes. Another one of my own vet's favorite recitations.

On one hand, I'm proud that I saved Sprout. But it came at a cost.

Some months later, he dropped her and several of their other pets off for boarding for a few days while he vacationed. She needed to update her vaccinations at the same time. Guess what? Sweet Sprout didn't exist for us anymore. At home, she was fine. In the clinic? Only the demonized version. She knew immediately where she was, and we were lucky to get her into the cat kennel at all. Guess what else? The owner called incessantly, worried about whether she had calmed down. I mean, multiple times every hour. We tried over and over again to explain it was better for us to *not* keep going in and out of the room to try to soothe her, but to leave the cat alone. We begged him not to worry about it and to just give her time. Plenty of our kitty boarders are angry the first day, but with a little grace, privacy, and time, most calm down. It's a lesson in patience. Often by day two, we can reach in and pet those same cats that were ready to bite the day prior.

He couldn't handle it. I'm sure it was ruining his short vacation for the rest of his family. In the end, I think they cut the trip short because he was so worried about the cat. She never did get her vaccines updated, between her attitude about the whole thing and the owner's never-ending calls. Sprout has never been back since. If they go on vacation anymore, I believe they learned their lesson and hire a cat-sitter to stop by the house.

Bittersweet victory.

Life & Death

"You can easily judge the character of a man by how
he treats those who can do nothing for him."
—Johann Wolfgang von Goethe

When you spend a great deal of time learning a certain trade, it's natural that you begin to view the world from the perspective of that particular lens. Veterinary medicine is no different. I have come to perceive the world, and people, based on their animal ownership.

Truly, I believe I see the best and the worst in people. It's a double-edged sword.

People come first. It's the unwritten rule of our society, and I'm not going to argue the point. I don't have the powers of debate to accomplish it. What I do believe is that humans are connected to the world we inhabit, and we are responsible for it. The earth, with all its flora and fauna. Showing disregard will only serve to hurt ourselves in the end. If you want the religious aspect, we ought to be good stewards of our planet. If religion is not your thing, just know that research concerning good welfare of other living organisms is continually linked to positive benefits for humans as well. Point is, whatever your reasoning, we can all agree on that. Take care of nature; it serves us, too.

Every kind of human owns animals. When one is completely responsible for the well-being of a living creature, true colors show.

Do they provide the basic necessities required? Do they do more, for the enrichment of the animal? Do they show affection towards them? What about when the burdensome parts of animal ownership come about?

It's easy for one to be a good steward, or a good owner, when things are going well. Alas, smooth seas don't make good sailors. Inevitably, there will be "burdensome" times. A problematic behavior. A stressful illness or accompanying symptom. An expensive veterinary bill.

I can promise you all veterinary staff are tired of hearing the joke by sticker-shocked owners. "Oh, wow. Too bad you can't claim dogs as a dependent, right?"

Yes, I know there's pet insurance out there. But as previously mentioned, I'm not a fucking salesman and I'm not going to regale anyone with the finer points of plans available. Most of my clients don't have pet insurance, and maybe that's the norm in some areas. For many, it's unrealistic. And no matter how you slice it, pet ownership is expensive.

Sometimes it takes heroic measures to try to save a pet from an illness or trauma of some kind. Guarantees of success will obviously vary case-by-case, but it's an important question to ask. And a very *fair* question to ask, especially if there's a hefty price tag. *If I consent to XYZ diagnostics or treatments for Cuddles, what are the possible outcomes?* If a poor prognosis is a factor, sometimes it's more about the worthiness of the recommended treatment, rather than the cost. Is it worth putting Cuddles through "all of that" at her age and condition? Also fair questions, with variable answers.

You're not a bad person for asking about the practicalities. If treatment is both doable and affordable, I hope you'd give them that chance.

For many, it's not in the cards, and money is unfortunately one of the biggest driving forces. No way around it. You're not automatically lumped into "Bad Person" category, though.

I will never fault anyone for having to be careful about a budget, because for fuck's sake, I've been there, too. Everyone has a budget, really. Just in different amounts. What I do often see is the irresponsible decision about owning the pet in the first place. Such as blowing the whole budget on the initial price tag of the pet—often easily into the thousands of dollars—and then having little left for health care and practical expenses. If you paid close attention to past chapters, you'll remember how I feel about breeders. I like mutts and rescues better, anyways. I'll also never pay anywhere near that amount to purchase a dog. Especially a breeder pup. I said what I said.

You haven't planned well if you have not budgeted for preventive care. We touched on those old life-saving vaccines and whatnot earlier in the parvo section. Or, to spay or neuter your animal. We're the ones who have seen pets die of preventable conditions, because they were never vaccinated or fixed. Spaying and neutering are about more than reducing the population, though that's damn important, too. Testicular cancers or diseases of the prostate. Mammary cancers, or the heartbreaking agony of pyometra, a deadly uterine infection.

Or, more simply than dealing with the high cost or inconvenience of pets, there's the rehoming trend. A popular scenario. Great choice especially for those who get a cat when their landlord said, "no pets" and hoping they won't notice. Tell me how fair that is to the animal, who had come to know that renter and their home as their own? Trusting in them. Only to be dumped or returned to the shelter when the landlord found out. Guys, they almost always find out. And when given the ultimatum of getting rid of the animal or moving out, I don't often hear of Sparky winning the battle. This is where bashing-head-against-wall frustration comes in for us. You selfish fucks.

But back to the point. Life and death.

There is usually no black-and-white answer for how to handle impending death. When a pet's time is winding down, barring acute and/or devastating illness or some other traumatic event, it's the natural order of things to just slow down. For age, senility, or the symptoms of organ failure and cancerous processes to creep in.

Owners often hope we'll tell them when the time is. They don't want to have to make that call. It's too hard. Too emotional. They wonder if they're calling it too soon, but they also don't want the pet to suffer. It's a broken record heard by veterinary staff, but I'm not upset when they ask. It shows their depth of caring. If the animal is suffering, and we think it would be kinder to say farewells sooner rather than later, we'll say so. But we are being honest when we say it's a subjective question. We know about the illness, but what we don't know is the pet. Not as well as they, the owner. And that's what I convey.

At what point does the bad outweigh the good? There are actual checklists one can find online to grade their animal's quality of life on a points system. Presumably more points equals a better quality of life, but you'd have to read the instructions. I will never hand an owner one of those charts, because it's cringey as fuck to make a decision as heavy as that, based on a math problem. Math was never my forte. But what I do appreciate about those checklists is getting the owner thinking about the subject matter. I ask them to consider how well the pet gets around. How difficult is it for them to perform their basic bodily functions? If that is still in place, then whether there is enjoyment. Does Jinx still enjoy the things he used to enjoy? Excitement for treats, playtime, or bonding snuggles …? Those are questions the owner can answer better than us.

I won't lie. Some do let things go further than we'd recommend. Often, we don't see patients during the illness process, until the owner has decided their time has come. Or, I have an owner right now that is a classic denier of how bad his dog looks. A big Lab, hardly able to stand anymore. Dyspneic, barely moving, barely eating. And as the veterinarian and I are exchanging knowing looks that it ought to be time, the owner's telling us how much progress the dog has made, since he got up and moved from one room to the next—for the first time in three days. So, he's certainly not ready to let him go. We had to have the easing-him-into-it conversation anyways, but in the meantime, sent home more pills to keep doggo comfortable in his remaining days.

Another very kind owner's dog passed away at home, but he didn't feel qualified to make that determination. He called, asking if he had time to bring the suspect-deceased dog into the clinic before I closed on my Saturday shift. I stayed late for him. When he laid the body on my exam table, it was extremely obvious. I suspect most Average Joes off the street would have recognized sweet Bonnie was gone. Stiff with rigor mortis, eyes vacant, and bearing the telltale scent. Still, the owner was uncertain, and so for his comfort, I pulled my stethoscope off the wall hanger. Listened attentively for an obligatory amount of time for Bonnie's heart or any movement of air through her lungs. Of course there was nothing to be heard on auscultation, but the owner appreciated that I took the time to confirm his sad news. There was nothing more I could do for Bonnie but prepare her body for the cremation with dignity.

Most of the time, owners have a decent gauge for when it's the right time. It's rare that I question it, if they feel they've reached that point. Nonetheless, if they need my reassurance they're doing the right thing, I can't think of a time I answered that question with anything but sincerity.

The only times I wouldn't say, "You're doing the right thing," is when the question is not being asked. The selfish assholes of the world. The elderly woman that wanted to put the old dog down because he was having urinary accidents, and they'd just recarpeted the house. Doggo was inconvenient, and who had time to bother with diagnostics? Or, the lady that dropped off the dog and didn't stay for the euthanasia with us, when I observed the hind leg had literally rotted off him. I wouldn't have blamed her, had she come in months earlier and said she couldn't afford or invest the time in treating a cancerous mass on the dog. Instead, she let it wait to a point of severe neglect.

It's rare that I opt to *not* send owners a sympathy card, but those might have been two notable exceptions.

—

People often say, "Oh, I could never do what you do. I couldn't stand to put animals down." Which is kind of a condescending thing to say, honestly, but I try not to think about it too much.

I know what they mean to say. They don't have the stomach for it. I have a very regular client who, when she sees the lit candle on our lobby counter, signifying a euthanasia is in progress, will 'nope' out of there and leave as fast as she can. Can't handle it. Doesn't want to see it. No accidental glimpses of the pets, nor other crying owners. It's too much for her.

We don't put animals down because it's pleasant for us. We do it because it's in their best interest, and because we've dedicated our professional selves and our lives to their care. So please be careful with *us* and how you phrase that observation about how you couldn't do what we do.

That said? The truth is, *euthanasia is not the hard part of the job.*

I don't mean to imply it's an enjoyable pastime. Of course not. But, it's not euthanasia that makes me lose sleep. What does? Neglect. Disregard. General callousness or dickishness. That's a different topic.

In another chapter, we talked about the word origin. In Greek, *euthanasia* means a "good death." And I believe in that as an option in the veterinary world. It's a kind service we can offer to pets. I mean it, whenever I tell that owner they're making the right decision. Euthanasia doesn't keep me awake at night. Nearly always, in their last moments, those pets are there with family members who loved them. It's bittersweet, knowing they're saying goodbye, but that heartbroken owner? Whether they're tearing up gracefully or bawling their eyes out, they're surrounding their animal with affectionate adoration. Realizing the heaviness of their loss as they reminisce on time they've spent with their pet.

I've been privileged to witness expressions of gratitude for the life of their companion. Declarations of love. Final pictures snapped. Sometimes, prayers are spoken over them. Snappy tributes. I'm not a great hugger, but I've given hugs when it's called for. Such as the client that didn't want their dachshund to be left in the exam room alone, even after she had passed. I've held a devastated woman who could hardly stand up, so distraught after losing most all her pets in a house fire. Yes, plenty of tears have been shed in that exam room. Some stiff upper lips, too, but then it's a lost cause by the time they reach the parking lot. Some swear they'll never get another, because how could they replace what they lost? Or, because it's so hard to lose them at all, and they're afraid of going through heartbreak again. Meanwhile, others immediately feel the need to fill their grief with new life.

One of my devastated clients left her beloved dog's euthanasia appointment and found someone in a parking lot, selling pups out of the back of their truck. Not even a block away. She didn't make it back home yet, before getting a new dog. Some will criticize that choice, but it's not for me to say. If her heart was capable of giving love to the next animal, who am I to judge? Who am I to question the serendipitous ways of the universe? We all grieve in our own way. I hope it worked out for her and the new puppy.

Another time, the rather large family group that came to attend the end-of-life appointment were taking turns going into the exam room. The young children went first to say their goodbyes. After, they stepped out with their father, while the mother and grandparents remained with the pet for the process. While I wasn't attempting to eavesdrop from where I sat behind the desk in our small lobby, I couldn't help but overhear the father's eloquent explanation of death to his crying daughter. The girl lamented that the beloved family pet couldn't live forever. In age-appropriate language, he told her how that made the dog's life even more of a gift. Like flowers, there is beauty in impermanence. Therefore, how much more cherished was the time they got to share with their beloved companion, because it couldn't last forever? I can normally remain stoic, but there may have been a lump in my throat on that one.

Some of them get to me, from time to time. I may shed a quiet tear or two. The truth is, we perform those appointments so often that I can't get too worked up about them. I'd fall apart in two weeks, if I did. My aim is to be respectful. To give the pet and the owners the dignity of a "good death" experience, to the best of my ability. The best it can be, in the circumstances. Sometimes I take the lead on being the gentle voice in the room, and sometimes there's another who pulls off the soothing role better than me. I can be supporting cast. No problem. But I am not usually weepy. It's not because I don't care. It's so I can continue serving the next new life cycle that comes in with a wagging tail.

For the Sake of Levity: Bears, Oh My!

My coworker, a brilliant RVT, was doubled over in laughter when she came out of the exam room. Face crimson, tears streaming down her cheeks, wheezing for breath. It was several moments before she could tell us what had earned such a reaction.

The medical notes probably sounded something like this:

Patient presented for teddy bear accidentally glued to fur. O unable to get it out.

I'll never know the how or the why. I'm just happy it happened.

Your Breedist Aunt

"The better I get to know men, the more I find myself loving dogs."
—Charles de Gaulle

If every family has that racist uncle they have to endure at Thanksgiving dinner, I might as well be the breedist aunt. You know what? Before you point your judgmental bird-finger my way, know this to be true. Working in a veterinary capacity has made breedists out of pretty much every single one of us. Some of us have different tolerances for certain types over others, but all cohorts I've worked with, which has been a decent number at this point, have their favorites and their not-so-favorites. If you're in the field and claim you haven't groaned aloud when you heard "Mrs. Smith is coming in with her *fill-in-the-blank-breed*," then I call you a straight-up liar. Or it's still your first week on the job. Hey, welcome.

You'll get there.

Most of us, too, have had our idealist breeds we always wanted to own, until we set foot in our practice roles. For me, I used to think I wanted a dachshund or a husky. Go ahead, vet friends. It's ok. You can laugh. We all have to learn sometimes, right?

When it comes to animal breeds, there's a reason for the stereotypes that come with them. We're talking medical and behavioral issues, both. Ignoring them, I think, is a foolish proposition.

As I touched on in a previous chapter about my darling Eggs Benedict, it's crucial for owners to understand the breed of animal they own, or intend to own. *What are they genetically designed for?*

Are they a working dog requiring significant stimulation to keep their intelligent mind active, rather than becoming destructive with no job to do? Consider your poor apartment couch cushions, and how you might feel to come home to find them ripped to shreds like a blanket of snow. Or, is it a herding dog, and yet you have no sheep but only a toddler who won't enjoy their ankles being nipped at? Consider how unfair it is on your family's legs: they just want to walk to the bathroom in peace. Are you thinking of taking a brachycephalic (smoosh-face) dog for five-mile jogs with you every day? Consider whether you have enough energy to both jog and carry said dog when it collapses from working so hard to breathe. Do you have time for that adrenaline-fueled hunting dog to burn mountains of energy all the time, or are you expecting it to lie still on a couch and therefore contain the brimming enthusiasm it has for life? Consider that it's not fair for you to yell at that dog for jumping on you in excitement, leaving foot-long angry red scratches on your skin, when it has no other outlet to exude its zest.

For a long time in the history of biological and psychological study, scientists argued over whether it was nature or nurture that made a person what they were. Were they born this way, hereditarily destined to become a product of their parents' genetic makeup? Or were they rather influenced by their environment as they grew up—the parenting style they experienced, the location of their childhood, their friends' attitudes, their impactful moments, et cetera? Well, enough theorists and scientists decided it wasn't just one or the other, but both, interplaying with each other.

The same is true for sentient animals. If you're not considering the breed-specific needs of your pet, it's going to harm both of you in the end.

Do your fucking research.

For a short period of time, I volunteered as a zoo docent at my local zoo. Most of our tasks revolved around helping with activity days for the public. Face-painting, rock-painting, animal-themed bowling, or bean-bag tosses, and that type of thing. Much of it was restraint or handling the animals available in the zoo education center. We had to be trained for all types of creatures there. Some slithered, some crawled, some squawked. Once you'd gotten through the training portion, you had a certain amount of freedom to pick your favorites that you could feature for a public event.

When it was my turn to go to the local mall to represent the zoo at an event day, the blue-tongued skink went with me. Pretty chill, liked a warm spot on your arm, and so slow-moving, people were fascinated when they realized it was a living creature. Not taxidermy. Back at the education center, though, my favorite snake was the Western hognose. He came with a little bit of an attitude. If you knew when and how to anticipate it, it wasn't bad at all. I learned to expect the strike from the little snake when his container was first opened. I refrained from flinching. Once that was over with, I could pick him up with ease. The retroussé snout, too adorable to pass up.

The coordinator of the education center had a regular saying for us, as a reminder to be careful and cautious with our handling technique, and for the public audience to follow the rules.

Anything with a mouth can bite.

It's the simplest of rules, but I find it's a good reminder for veterinary environments as well. Especially where animals may be in pain or afraid. It may not be their normal behavior at home. But if they possess a mouth, they can bite. A prime example was an elderly couple with their two fat Pomeranians. Both of them perfectly nice dogs. Never had a behavior problem. Just needed the frequent reminders the dogs were overfed and could stand to lose some weight. I mean, they were practically sphere-shaped. Veterinary friends here won't be shocked to know one had a collapsing trachea and probably Pickwickian syndrome, besides a bad heart. I won't forget the final time they brought the older one in on a Saturday morning, stating he seemed to be having a little bit of a hard time catching his breath. They hoped to pass him off for a quick fix while they ran some errands and come back for him.

They handed him to me across the lobby desk. His tongue was as blue as my blue-tongued skink. That normally nice Pomeranian suddenly bit my hand, because of the awkward pass-off and his positionally-dependent ability to breathe. He panicked. I have exercise-induced asthma, so I have a notion of how terrifying it is to feel like you're gasping for oxygen through a straw. I can't blame the Pom, but the bite still hurt. Didn't break the skin, so I kept it to myself as the doctor briefly looked and we both came to the same conclusion. He didn't mince words. No time for them to run errands. The wife stayed for that euthanasia, but the husband was so upset he couldn't speak and had to go outside. They tried harder to get the weight down on the second Pom after that. It's still a struggle, but the effort is there. Old habits.

Pomeranians weren't a big one on my stand-out list for deserved stereotypes. We might as well dive into the offensive subject.

In my personal experience, I can honestly say there's only one breed of dog that I've encountered consistently that is *always* a nice dog. Like, I've never met a mean one. Even if they were uncomfortable or in pain, I can't conceive of one trying to bite. I won't say never, but it's hard to imagine. The Cavalier King Charles spaniel. Truly, if anyone out there can say otherwise, I'll be fascinated to find out. And how fitting for a dog with adorably dopey almond-shaped eyes, a button nose, and fluffy ears that looks like it should model a baby fashion line of clothing. That said, there's always a trade-off. A King Charles may earn an above-average rating for congeniality points, but they're a train wreck for health problems. Notorious for eye issues, bad hearts, hip dysplasia, luxating patellae, ear infections, and even some neurologic syndromes, any owner of this cute breed can expect to drop some money to keep them in good shape.

What other breeds can cause one to anticipate expense? Basically, any brachycephalic. Bulldogs especially. English bulldogs, Old English bulldogs, French bulldogs, even American bulldogs. Boston terriers. Pugs. Shih tzus, Pekingese, Lhasa apsos, Shar Peis, Brussels griffons. Sometimes boxers, too. My bulldog-loving clients have heard my veterinarian joke many times they'll be putting his kids through college if they keep buying the breed. They're known for the obvious trait of their smooshed snout with all its skin folds. The short snub-nose. That's what brachycephalic means, after all. A *shortened head*. And it's the feature that attracts most of those owners. They think the flat face is cute. Most of them come to learn that anatomical structure comes at the cost of their airway being compromised. Due to a few reasons. Stenotic nares, for instance, where the nostril openings are way too narrow. I recall inadvertently making one of my poor assistants feel bad when she brought a new pug puppy to see me and the doctor in the back room. She simply thought Puppy was cute and wanted to show her off, thinking we'd gush over her, too. Both the doctor and I took one look at her and responded with something more along the lines of, "Jesus Christ, why? Ugh! That poor nose! Fuck."

It's hard not to be frustrated by the bad breeding of these dogs. Like the Pomeranian, brachycephalics can be prone to problems with weak cartilage of their larynx or trachea, causing either of them to collapse and requiring extra effort to open back up for good airflow. Sometimes they can have a trachea smaller than normal. In some cases, an extended bony process past the dog's pharynx can cause obstruction to their airway. And, quite commonly, many brachycephalic breeds have an elongated palate. Basically, the roof of their mouth is too long and can cause partial blockage to the trachea. Honestly, these are just some of the breathing issues. It can get more complicated. These dogs are the ones snorting and breathing loudly, snoring like crazy. Getting overheated can do them in. Bulldog owners have to be careful about overexercising them. If we ever have them under anesthesia, which they tend to be high risk patients for, we joke they've never breathed so well as when there's an endotracheal tube feeding them oxygen. Once it's time for that tube to be removed, back to the snorting gasp for dear life.

Besides the breathing issues, these breeds are notorious for bad skin. I've seen my doctor try to get away with abbreviating his medical notes to just say "bulldog skin" for a diagnosis. Masses of skin folds don't help. Creases and crevices like to harbor moisture. Bacteria, dermatitis, allergies, or fungal lesions can be rampant. Ear infections galore. Wait, there's more! Elbow dysplasia, spinal abnormalities, dental chaos, dystocia or even a complete inability to give birth without a C-section, digestive concerns, eye problems ... I mean, the list is frankly never-ending, and most of these things are chronic. One vet visit isn't going to cure any of it. Be prepared to be a frequent flyer if you want to keep your bulldog's issues to a dull roar. I wish we had reward punch cards to offer you.

Oh, if we want to poke fun at me next, let's add dachshunds to the list. They're one of the breeds that has potential to be a very sweet, cuddly dog, or a complete jackass. But if you do get a nice one, guess what comes with that elongated body? If you said anything related to back problems, ding-ding, gold star for you! That spine is high risk for genetic defects or proneness to injury. All it takes is one misstep for the cute little sausage jumping off the Ottoman, and then you're rushing him in for steroids or anti-inflammatories because he can't walk. Enjoy those long weeks of strict cage rest, or expensive surgeries to get him back on track. Besides the touchy spinal areas, you can expect a dachshund to be a sewer mouth if they're over the age of six and have not had dental work yet. It's a lot of teeth cramped into a small orifice. If I've got a dachshund dental on the books that's not had the procedure for a few years, or ever, I ask for a wide berth surrounding that appointment slot. We're about to have a field day of extractions. The last point of note I'll make in their case? While any animal has the potential to ingest something they shouldn't, our little wiener friends are frequent offenders. That's not scientific analysis, but personal observation. I have restrained dachshunds enduring enemas or invasive rectal procedures to extract foreign material clogging up their exit. Notably, bathroom trash. Discarded tissues and feminine hygiene products are irresistible to these dogs. The more you've left your own bodily goo, the more they want it. Yum. Other dachshunds have had the misfortune to be obstructed by their foreign material of choice and require surgical extraction from the GI tract. You've been warned. Keep a lid on the bathroom can that, to a dachshund, sings a song of sweet serenade.

And for my other offense, the Siberian husky. If you don't own one, you probably think they look majestic. From a distance, they do. But let's be honest. It wasn't the host of eye issues they're prone to acquiring that made me change my mind. It's the high anxiety and a drama queen attitude. Just look at one wrong and you're probably going to be cleaning up blowout diarrhea. Multiple times. They're nervous as fuck and most of the owners I've seen don't do enough to keep them properly exercised. When they're not exercised, the husky's propensity for nerves and anxiety increases. Most were not mean, though we've had a small few that won't be handled. But you can expect dramatic whining and howling if they're asked to obey any command they don't feel like doing. You'd think I was stabbing them with a knife when all I did was coax them onto the exam table. Nope. No thank you. Pass on ownership of these majestic cry-babies.

There's not necessarily anything wrong with the majority of them, but do know I roll my eyes at your designer breeds of dog. Shorkies and schnorkies and morkies and schnoodles and whatever else. It also gives us a little bit of a thrill to write "mixed" under the breed description on our file, after you've paid an absurd fortune for your mutt.

Now, Doodles on the other hand? I'll be honest—when have I not? I think they're cute puppies, but straight-up strange looking dogs when they grow to adulthood. I don't get the appeal. If you love these mutts, and yes, they're mutts, not purebred, just know that even the "inventor" of these dogs regrets what he's done. Whether you got the golden retriever-poodle version or the Labrador-poodle model, you tend to get the worst of each breed in your mixture. I'll say they're usually nice dogs, but there's not much more. They're high-anxiety in their temperaments and the health problems should make them a non-starter for continuance of existence. It's another breed at risk for severe hip dysplasia, bad skin, ear infections, Addison's disease, epilepsy, thyroid disorders, heart conditions, and a list of eye conditions as well. Cute.

If you're anticipating whether I'll talk about vicious dogs or trigger your anger over it, here you go. Let's get to the controversial part.

First, with the helpful reminder of my zoo education coordinator. *Anything with a mouth can bite.*

There. So. No matter the size, anything with claws and teeth has the capability of using them. We take biters seriously, and I have no patience for anyone who thinks it's funny when a small dog bites. Yes, I've met people that try to laugh it off. Guess what? It still hurts. I had just the very tip of my finger bitten by a shih tzu when I was giving an oral vaccine. (That's what I get for letting a doctor restrain him. Ha. A good technician would have done better. Yeah, I said it.) That fingertip hurt for months afterwards. Thankfully that's all it was. And speaking of shih tzus, one of my client families was new in town and going to transfer all their previous vet records over. I got a nervous feeling in my stomach when I realized they owned two massive Akitas. A breed notorious for viciousness, and I'd already heard horror stories, including a family's toddler nearly being scalped by one and only the owner severely beating it with a baseball bat made the dog let go of the child. So, imagine my surprise when I received the reports for the Akitas and saw no marked behavior concerns, until the third pet. Their shih tzu, less than a year old, was absolutely ferocious. Untouchable. And yet the Akitas were manageable. You never know.

Chow Chows are just a no-no. In my memory, the first time I ever saw one was as a fresh veterinary assistant. His arrival was announced with squeals of delight by the other female staff. When the puppy plodded in, I could see the appeal. Like a furry bear cub, it was kind of adorable. They gathered around him, cooing and petting him in excitement, and he responded with a good demeanor. And that's about the last good thing I could say for the breed. The few adult Chow Chows we ever tried to examine besides that puppy couldn't be touched. I remember vividly, a patient had injured himself and was unable to walk. The owners were worried about getting the dog into the building and called when they arrived, asking for help. Well, I and the other assistant served only to be decoration after passing off the stretcher to the owners. That enormous bear of a dog wouldn't allow us near him, and I decided I comfortably preferred to keep my limbs intact. Owners had to do all the lifting and handling themselves. At my most recent clinic, I felt a little bad when a potential client came in holding a dog at the end of her leash. Sitting behind the tall lobby desk, I was unable to see what the creature was. She asked to schedule a grooming appointment, and I launched into the lengthy description of drop-off times, required vaccines, and options for grooming services. We were well into it before the doctor wandered through and saw what dog was at the desk, out of my sight. He stopped me. It wasn't a rude dismissal, but he was very frank with the young lady. We wouldn't be taking the appointment, as we no longer see Chows. Even our groomer, who is someone I exalt as having the patience of a saint with difficult dogs, drew a line with that breed. The doctor had already banned them after having nearly been mauled by one himself. A naïve owner had once brought one in, swearing Chow Chow was sweet as could be. The moment the dog was touched in the exam room, it went berserk, lunging, snarling, and trying to bite. The doctor was able to keep him at bay by having the leash wrapped around the other side of the table. Meanwhile, the terrified owner had bolted out the door, not realizing what doggo was capable of until that moment. Not so sugar and spice as he thought.

I suppose it's fair to alternate sizes and go back to a smaller demon. A frequent offender of the Napoleon complex is our friend, the Chihuahua. I've owned one myself, against my better judgement. And even though mine had a front leg deformity, in which his paw resembled a lobster-claw, I made absolutely sure that dog walked of his own volition the majority of the time. He was capable. I only carried him in his advanced age when his arthritis tired him out during walks. I won't have a purse-dog mentality in my home. When small dogs are held all the time, they tend to think they are as big as the height at which they're held, so they'll have no qualms about challenging something significantly bigger than they are. Additionally, because they're small, owners tend to think it's funny and don't correct the bad behavior. If you would tell a big dog "No!" for an undesirable behavior, it should be the same for your small fry. My own Chihuahua loved people. Adored them, actually. He would be content to sit in anyone's lap if they would care to pet him. But true to his breed, he would try to start something with any other dog. Didn't matter if they were ten times his size. He was reprimanded, even if it was sometimes funny.

I guess the difference between my little ankle biter and a big dog that's mean is simply that one's easier to handle. If I've got a demon Chihuahua for a patient —and believe me, I've seen some hellions—I can out-muscle them. Or get a bulky towel around them to prevent myself and other staff from a sharp bite. Stop them from out-maneuvering me by smothering their limbs with my shield. As for the bigger dogs? I can't always win those battles, if muscle is required. The bigger or stronger the dog with an attitude, the more dangerous they are, and the more likely we'll turn them away as a patient. If you've got a mean Great Dane, it's not worth me getting injured, nor any staff. I can't restrain that, and I won't try. I once brought an estimate to a Great Dane owner for sedation so we could do an effective ear cleaning, as our strategy of having two or three staff hold doggo against a wall while another one performed the procedure was still too difficult. She balked at the cost, and that was that. Her rude response didn't inspire us to keep trying to help. Take doggo home and do it yourself. If we can see the problem and just send home medications, we may opt to try that. But if the owner can't step up and handle their own pet at home, we can't always promise we'll do it for you at the clinic either. Not without drugs.

My mother and I have both been bitten by Dalmatians. I was a young kid riding my bicycle down our suburban street when I pedaled past a neighbor's house with one loose in the front yard. I slowed down my bike when I noticed her approaching me. "She's friendly, don't worry about Leika!" the lady promised.

Leika then jumped up and bit me in the side, drawing blood and ripping a hole in my tie-dye monkey shirt. I don't recall an apology of any kind, but hopefully they kept better control when the next child went by. A few years later, during a walk, my mother noticed a different Dalmation stuck in the ditch. I couldn't say what the dog got stuck on. Maybe he got trapped in trash or was sinking into mud on that drizzly day. But he was frightened and my mother tried to go down to help. It's a difficult thing when you're still a child to see your parent cry, and I'll never forget my mother bursting into the kitchen after that episode, gasping through tears of pain with her hand torn open and bleeding. She drove herself to the urgent care clinic while I was left to deal with the animal control officers. Shaken, I couldn't answer their questions straight when they asked me which of my mother's hands bore the injury. But I recall being present when they and the dog-sitter of that Dalmation had to fetch him from the ditch down the street from where we lived. I'd begged the dog-sitter to be careful, to not go down there after seeing what happened to my mother. I was a pre-teen kid then, but she took my advice, calling to the dog from afar, also scared to approach until the officer arrived. Clearly the dog had escaped the yard. I wondered how that conversation went when they called to tell the actual owner of the series of events and mandated quarantine period. Years later, my mother still has a vivid scar from the incident. When you're a kid, you always see a Dalmation depicted as the best friend of firemen, and there's the Disney film featuring a hundred-and-one of those dogs, which makes you think they're cuddly. To be fair, I've not seen many in practice. They're not as popular a breed as they once were. But they do scare me, and especially when the few I have seen are poorly behaved. Only two or three very good Dalmatians have come across my path, who had owners with better-than-average awareness of behavioral practices. One was a coworker. Apart from those exceptions, I'll admit to my bias against the spotted canines.

Heelers? I live in a place where they're popular. As a herding dog, they're meant to be out working on their country property. Again in fairness, I think with a lot of my clients, that's exactly what they do. Props. But they're not much accustomed to coming into town. Or at least, they don't act like it when they get to our clinic. They're terrified, skittish, and most of them would gladly bite you from fear. Seeing a nice one is a rare, notable exception. To the point that when it does occur, that's all we have to say.

"Ugh. Great. A 4:30 p.m. heeler vaccine appointment?"

"Yeah, but it's the nice one! Remember Daisy?"

"Oh, yeah the *good* one! Thank God!"

Border collies are up there, too, but in my experience, have tended to be even more aggressive to people than their heeler cousins. We've asked several border collie patients not to be brought back, because when they're fractious, they're too quick to handle. Big enough to do some damage. Not much more to say about them, so we'll keep it moving.

Shepherds? Similar story. Take a heeler's fearful skittishness, blended with husky-like anxiety. It's a hot mix with a full-on willingness to bite the shit out of you. In contrast to heeler owners, I don't know what it is about shepherd breeds, but the wrong people want to own them. I wish there was a nicer way to say that, but it's usually someone who just likes the aesthetic of a shepherd. Unfortunately, most are not equipped to handle them. They have a poor grasp of how much these intelligent, working dogs require stimulation and experienced care. German shepherds, Australian shepherds, and Anatolian shepherds are some of the ones I see. So many of them, badly socialized. And those are large, powerful dogs to not have manners.

We've had sketchy encounters with GSDs (German shepherd dogs) that leave us not wanting to get too close to some of them. I witnessed an inexperienced VA make the split-second mistake of reaching for a fractious shepherd that had gotten loose in the treatment area. In a flash, he snapped and tore her fingers open. Almost certainly, she needed a surgical fix. I never saw her return to work. The owner of that dog later elected to euthanize, due to its aggression and an increasing list of incidents and offenses.

One of our patients was owned by a spouse who died, and the surviving owner was left with a temperamental shepherd that's since had a small fortune dropped onto him, trying to find trainers and boarders who can handle him, and regular therapy of Prozac to keep him manageable. One boarding vet facility told the client they would never keep him again after a disastrous attempt that required the client to cut their vacation short to come home and get the dog. Client started coming to my clinic afterwards. Not because we promised we could board the dog any better. In fact, we told the client we wouldn't keep him either. But because we took time to tactfully explain the difficulties with the dog, they were happier with us. Still, once a year we all get nervous when it's time for the German shepherd's appointment. The owner ups his dose and we dance around like sprites on a sugar high, distracting him with peanut butter and sing-songy voices just long enough to jab some vaccines into him and then get him back out the door. Does he get a thorough exam? Hell no. Because he's out of control and it's not worth us getting hurt over him. The owner understands that. They're just glad someone will see the dog at all. On a health note? I'll mention it seems to be more common to find poor specimens among GSDs. We've had some terrible breeders in our vicinity, and some of those dogs, even the young ones, have come in hardly able to walk on their rear legs. Already predisposed to hip and elbow dysplasia and degenerative myelopathy, they got dealt heavier doses of the conditions.

As for those Aussies? They're stupidly popular right now, and I hate it. We've had more incidents with Aussies than any other breed lately. They snap, and most dangerous of all, they do it without warning. For any mathematicians sitting there saying, well, duh. If you see more of a certain breed, you're going to see a higher ratio of problematic ones … Yeah, I take that point. But the vast majority of them are difficult. I should be able to talk about a decent percentage of lovability and sweetness. Instead, I can hardly conjure any examples in my head. Maybe two. That's the truth. For whatever reason, they've caught on as a breed everyone wants to have, but few people should. We saw one recently for a urinary problem. The assistant was able to take him outside and get a sample for me to run. Sometimes sticking a bowl underneath a dog makes them nervous, but the VA obtained it. Dog went back inside for its exam. The vet did his whole look-over while talking to the owner, head-to-tail. At the last minute, he remembered he'd done everything but heart and lung auscultation. He grabbed his stethoscope and held the device against the dog's chest to listen. And that was it. With no growl, no whine, no warning of any kind, the dog whipped around and bit him in a flash. Just like my mother's episode with the Dalmation, I went into our clinic kitchenette to find the doctor washing a bloodied hand with severe gashes on his wrist and fingers.

Another Aussie came for a vaccine update. The first adult set. The owner fumbled getting the muzzle on the sketchy dog, and we were doomed after that. Knowing what was coming, none of the staff, myself included, could safely apply a muzzle to the animal. Snapping jaws, whipping his aggressive head, and lunging. We tried several tactics, with the owner trying to talk to him soothingly and also having her leave the room. She finally got tired of watching us try out in the empty lobby. She picked up the leash and left without another word and no part of the exam completed. I never knew if she was embarrassed at the dog's behavior or fed up with our inability. Never heard from her again. In contrast, I have another Aussie patient we were able to muzzle, and if you were permitted to read my notes in the health chart, you would find my description of having to use my whole body to pin him against the exam table for seconds while the doctor hurried to vaccinate him before we released him. I've also helped on cases where we euthanized them, not due to age or any health condition, but due to their fractiousness. One, a perfectly healthy young dog, less than two years old. But she had traumatized her family and was completely untrustworthy around anyone else. L-i-a-b-i-l-i-t-y. After multiple incidents, the father came to the decision and scheduled the appointment with us. He came alone. Asked us not to send a sympathy card or anything, as he was telling the kids he'd rehomed her. Truth is, rehoming a dog like that is extremely difficult. You can't in good conscience give them to someone else, unless you know they have expertise in such cases. That's a rare find, and we supported his decision. Well, not the dishonesty to the family part. But the decision his animal was unsafe and holding the family's lives hostage by tiptoeing around her vicious tendencies. That's not an ok situation for anyone.

Pitbulls.

The current breed in the spotlight of controversy. If you're a pitbull apologist, I imagine this is the section you've been looking for. To see where I stand. Will we be in solidarity, or will I piss you off and make you throw this book in the gutter in a fit of indignant rage? Guess we'll see.

Pitbull is a general term that can include American bullies, American pit bull terriers, and Staffordshire bull terriers, among others. I've heard of some owners encouraged to be deceptive with usage of those names, to avoid saying they had a pitbull in a pitbull-sensitive location. "Call it a Staffordshire terrier, and they'll never know!"

Whatever you call them, I'm going to go back to origins. You shouldn't be surprised I want to consider nature and nurture. The breed has a complex and convoluted history. I won't go into excruciating depth, but it's worth noting what the pitbull's ancestors were designed to do. That muscular, stocky head wasn't for aesthetics, nor was the strong build. They were bred for cruel bloodsport. Literally, to taunt bulls to the point of exhaustion for the entertainment of spectators. Bulls, people. Think about the powerhouse of a dog required to take on such a task. Later, the breed was adapted a little more to take on the trend of "ratting." Competitors seeing whose dog could kill the most rats in an enclosed pen. Cute, right? And then that developed into actual dog fighting. The owners of those fighting dogs did want their pits to be loyal dogs to their humans, so that was a trait encouraged. Meanwhile, though, so was aggression towards other animals. The years of dog fighting waxed and waned. Obviously, such cruel practices are illegal now, but we've heard of it still happening here and there. Conversely, there were also trending periods in history where families found the breed a good companion in their home with their family, due to their loyal tendencies. Some of us have heard of pits as the "nanny" dogs for children.

With history in mind, let's turn to environment. Let's get my spoiler message in here, too. I've seen the sweetest pitbulls in the world, who come into my clinic excited to be petted, with wagging tails and eagerness for treats. Good dogs that seem like they could perfectly fit the "nanny" bill and be the loving image their advocates promote. I also see the polar opposite. And maybe it's that I live where I do, but I have a huge number of clients desiring and encouraging that aggressive trait. Leaving dogs intact rather than neutering, which might have reduced the potential aggression. Many who want the ear-cropped, tough-looking status symbol. Or as a guard for their property. Others just get saddled with the temperament and don't know what to do with it.

My own grandmother, states away, earned the nickname "Pitbull Wrestler" by the family. Out walking her Pomeranian one afternoon, the two were suddenly charged by a loose pit in the neighborhood. Not interested in Grammy, thankfully, however the pit was intent on killing her Pom. From miraculous pure adrenaline, Grammy yanked them apart and escaped. Pom was rushed to the emergency vet. The little dog survived the encounter, but not before losing an eye.

One of our older vets used to do ear-cropping for many years, and for many breeds. Pitbulls were up there, though. And while he was good at the procedure, he will tell you now he got tired of the type of clients who often requested it. It was the *only* thing they requested. To make their dog "look evil and shit," but couldn't be bothered with vaccines, fecal exams or dewormers, spaying or neutering. And as the practice began to fall out of favor, he decided he wouldn't miss doing it, either. He's given up those scissors gladly.

Whichever reason is behind the owner's aggressive pet, intention or circumstance, I respect the animal and what they are capable of. What they were originally bred for. Pitbulls get the rap that they do because they do have the power to kill. Both humans and other animals. Yes, I've had plenty of sweet-tempered ones deserving of jolly belly-rubs. I can also say I've had pitbull patients whose dispositions terrify me, with good reason.

I had a sick pit once that was going to require hospitalization. The young girl brought him in on a vicious looking chain, and I saw at once how he followed my every move with his eyes. I asked her from the get-go if the dog was ok to handle and approach.

"Oh yes," she said. "He won't attack you until I give the command to."

Comforting. A dog that could rip my throat out with ease. I approached with caution and care every time I went to his kennel. The veterinarian thought I was crazy and didn't dare get as close as I did. I felt the dog and I had an understanding, as long as I moved with slow purpose and spoke to him in his human family's native language. Low and gentle tones. Never acting excitable. Maybe that was foolish of me. Thankfully the dog was eventually discharged without incident.

I was in an adjacent room at one facility when another vet tech was mauled by a pit-mix. Gashing a deep wound to her head and tearing open her arm. She might have bled to death, had she been alone. Thank God someone else had been there to pull the leashed animal off her. The dog appeared quite content with itself up to the point of being euthanized an hour later, after she'd been taken away in an ambulance. His head still covered in her blood. This was an incident that left me traumatized, and even years later, invokes an emotional reaction.

We've euthanized several others for aggression, like the Aussies. Our vet gets unhinged when he hears of clients wanting to breed their bullies, for how sweet or pretty they are, or because their third cousin wants a puppy. Animal shelters are full of pits and pit-mixes that can't find homes. Your cousin might want one, but the other six or nine puppies still need homes, and good luck finding that many. Many get dumped, and pits are currently one of the most common breeds found in shelters. Slated for a life of confinement or eventual euthanasia when they remain unwanted.

One of my recent ones was the pet of a nice person who was utterly clueless. He'd done a kind deed, going to a dying relative's house out-of-state. Came back with an elderly intact pitbull the family member could no longer care for. It was clear that this was a dog left out in the yard and fed a terrible diet, with no vet care in its life. Similar to that Aussie we mentioned, the vet and I were able to handle the old boy when we started. He got onto the exam table nicely. Let us look over everything. The owner was gung-ho about wanting to fix him up and eagerly approved of the vet's recommendations for the works of preventive care. She suggested we start with the heartworm test. Only a drop of blood was needed. This vet is fond of the lateral saphenous vein to draw blood—a vein usually easy to access on the outside of a dog's back leg. And notably further away from the biting side of the animal. Good instinct, as it turned out. I held the vein ready for her, and as she poked with a baby twenty-five-gauge needle, a switch was flipped. The sweet old pitbull growled low, thank God, and that half second of warning was enough for me to urge her to get away. She did, leaping backwards just as he turned and snapped with vicious intent. Teeth baring and snarling. In a panic, the vet told me to let go. In my position, I felt that would be the bigger mistake. I had a side hold of the dog and enough of his collar so it would have been difficult for him to reach me, so I stayed put. I held on, and we managed to put a muzzle on him, vaccinated with great speed as the growling and snarling continued, and then called it done. Dewormer and heartworm test notions abandoned. Not worth it. And the owner, bless him, had no inkling of how dangerous a display his new-to-him dog had just put on. He'd assumed it to be run-of-the-mill. We had to explain to him over the course of subsequent requests for follow-up care that we were uncomfortable about his pet.

He came back about a month later for a sick visit. We got the pit on the table. Any attempt to palpate his stomach was met with that same response. And I nearly bit the vet myself for daring to try to lift up his tail to assess his rectum and think about obtaining a temperature. Intact male dogs tend to be particularly sensitive around that area. He wasn't having it.

They claimed he was a good dog around their family, but we continued to worry one wrong move would result in someone getting hurt. That dog had never been trained or made to do anything he didn't want to do. It would take very little to set him off. It may sound harsh, but we were relieved when its age and health caught up with him soon after, and they made the euthanasia appointment.

Bottom line? If brought up in a caring, experienced environment, yes, they have the potential to be great dogs. But I have no patience for people advocating for them with blanket statements about how they're all good and can do no wrong. Pit breeds were designed for dangerous work and they have equally dangerous ability. To ignore that fact is idiocy. To assume the humans that own them all have pure intentions, or are even knowledgeable about them, is a mistake. They are a breed that must be handled with understanding, love, and respect for their traits, good and bad.

Now, I've rambled long enough about dogs that it seems only fair I finish with a cat. Honestly, I can't claim we see a huge variety of different cat breeds. If we do, I'm less familiar with them. A couple of Minuets. A Persian. The occasional Maine coon. Maybe a few others, but most get assigned the typical domestic short/medium/long-hair on their breed description. Cats are cats, as far as disposition. Some are cooperative and friendly. Some very much aren't. And you'll remember my vet's fond saying, "Cats live and die by their own rules." But I will share about one cat breed we saw twice and will not bother with anymore.

Bengals. Truly, I don't know who thinks they make good pets, but Bengal cats are unmanageable. We were barely able to get an injection of sedative into the one dropped off to be neutered and could only watch as the long-legged feline jumped onto the impressive heights of our exam room shelves, over to the vaccine fridge, then spectacularly crash into the window in an effort to get outside. Knocking everything to the floor in his wake. We just waited for the drugs to take effect so we could get the procedure done and then put him safely away. Another client tried to bring theirs for a nail trim during our pandemic curbside service. We only got so far as touching the zipper to slightly open the crate, before deciding "nope" to the dilated eyes, huge teeth, and hissing tuna breath. I carried the crate back to the car and handed back the credit card that had no charges added to it. Cat bites have the potential to become dangerously infected. I've known vets put out of commission and hospitalized while recovering from cat bite complications. It's not worth it.

If we can avoid injuries to be able to return the next day to treat more pets, we'll choose that route. We reserve the right to refuse to see a patient that's too dangerous. Choose a pet you can handle, because it's not guaranteed we'll do it for you. One that you have proper time and facility to care for.

Know Thy Patient

"There may be medical tools in your hands to treat the patient, but those hands must be that of a loving, warm, and conscientious human being."
—Abhijit Naskar, *Time to Save Medicine*

Attention to detail. As I mentioned before, it's what I look for from good help. Someone who has an intuitive sense for their patients. An observant nature. It's a hard thing to teach. I mean, I can coach them on signs and symptoms to look for in a patient. How to be neat and orderly in preparing surgery packs. How to log the controlled substances correctly or take respectable medical notes. *What* to watch for can be learned. But it sure as fuck helps more if you're that person, by nature.

My mother worried about me in my formative childhood years. I assume most mothers worry in some sense or another about their offspring, but in my case, it was due to the fact that I never talked. Or, I wasn't talking when I was supposed to be. She would encourage me in every way she could think of. Attempt to make me repeat the words she was saying. Make me truly ask for the item I wanted when I was damn well old enough to ask. I refused.

"Juice? Do you want some juice? Yes, say *juice*, please!?"

She was already saying it for me. Why did I need to repeat? Yeah, I wanted juice. So I'd nod my head in the affirmative, ignore the superfluous requests for speech, and eventually she'd give in and surrender the juice so I didn't die of thirst.

I was a quiet baby, she always told me. Studying the world around me. Content to sit and watch the action, once my neck was strong enough to support my absurdly fat cheeks.

Still, my mother worried I might be stunted in some developmental way. Concerned I'd let my more gregarious little sister speak for me. And she would. A year apart in age, she would talk to anyone. Sing, dance, tell a stranger she loved them, whatever. And tell folks what her older sister wanted. Somehow she knew.

"I want the red popsicle, and she wants the purple one."

I'd nod. Yes. The purple was exactly the one.

I guess one day my little sister was busy. Or I just felt I could handle the situation. Couldn't say, as I have little memory of it myself. But the story goes that I approached my mother and out came the full sentence. No monosyllabic baby steps leading up to bigger words. No incoherent noises.

"Mama, can I have some juice, please?" I asked, clearly enunciating the request to the stunned woman.

Well, I can't explain to you today why I didn't bother talking as a toddler. My suspicion is that I haven't changed much. Maturity requires that I speak when appropriate. With the right people, hey, maybe I even enjoy it sometimes. Other times, I must pretend to be more outgoing than I am, and by the end of the night I'm exhausted. By nature? I'm fine shutting up. Observing. Sitting still and watching what a bird does in my backyard for fifteen minutes straight. Going on a hike that doesn't involve chatter with my hiking partner, just silent appreciation for the landscape. Listening to the conversations around me at Saturday night poker rather than chiming in, until it's necessary.

It's observation that makes one go the extra mile for their patients. A wise vet tech teacher of mine ranted to the class one day out of frustration. "I can teach you how to look at your lab results, but I can't teach you how to be compassionate, or to pay attention. How to be the person who says, 'when I feel sick, a warm bath makes me feel better, so I thought it might be nice to wipe my lethargic patient's face with a damp washcloth.' That just has to be your nature!"

I'm not the shiny face of the clinic, and I don't want to be. But if I've ever had a client be grateful to me personally, it's usually because I paid attention to their pet. Or I fought for their case.

In one incident, the thing any boarding facility hopes will never happen, happened. The worst. The boarding pet died, while we were watching him.

If an animal is quite elderly, we always worry about having them stay with us while the owner is out of town. In this case, we'll call the ancient Pomeranian-mix Poppy. The thing was, when it came to Poppy's death, the owner was grateful to me, in the end.

Why? For the simple fact that I paid attention. Don't misunderstand me, she was still heartbroken. But grateful. With the owner out of the state for a couple of weeks, we had time to get to know the two dogs she left.

That's the nature of boarding. Any good caretakers pick up quickly on the personalities of the pets. What works best for them individually. If they jump all over you in excitement or try to pee on your leg. If they lose their cool when the delivery truck rolls down the street. If they gobble their food or bury it in their blanket for safekeeping. One of my patients is a basset-corgi-mix that will tear any towel, blanket, sheet, or pillow to shreds. He'll even destroy the hard plastic grate in the kennel, chewing it apart, bit by bit. The only item safe in his presence is a polar bear stuffed animal, similar in form to a Beanie Baby. Loves it. Cherishes it. Somehow that fragile toy is intact, albeit slobbered-on. Only it is safe from demise.

But in Poppy's case, he was just a sweet little dog. No great trouble, except the occasional tiny accident on his towel. Old dog bladder. Easy to swap the soiled one out for a clean towel. I firmly believe in dogs being leash-trained, but Poppy was one of the rare exceptions I carried until I could place him gently into the grass. He was so frail. Could have been held in one hand. A bow-legged walk with his arthritic joints. Barely a tooth left in his head; nothing to hold in his ever-projecting tongue. Alopecic, fragile coat of hair remaining, but bright eyed and mobile.

One afternoon, a few days before the owner was due to return, I went to Poppy's kennel to get him out for his walk. Something wasn't right.

To this day, I couldn't tell you what it was that tipped me off. Nothing he was *doing* was different. His eyes weren't glazed over. He wasn't laterally recumbent or anything. No clue. I only knew that, after observing his mannerisms for several days, suddenly he carried himself strangely, for Poppy. He was … off. Nor did it improve when I set him on the grass.

It just wasn't *Poppy*.

I took him back inside and plopped him on the exam table. Took his temperature and was dismayed to find it terribly low. Auscultation of his heart revealed a bradycardic beat. I shouted for the veterinarian and after a more thorough look, he agreed with my assessment. Body systems seemed to be shutting down. The ancient Pomeranian-mix was apparently dying.

We deliberated for only a minute about whether to call the owner. I hate calling someone far away and helpless to do anything, causing them stress and worry on their vacation. Alas, *not* calling her would be worse. Catastrophic, if something did happen.

I didn't ask the doctor to do it. I did it myself. Got ahold of the lady and told her I was sorry to be bothering her on her trip, but I was worried about Poppy. Something wasn't right, and we were doing what we could to keep him comfortable. Encouraging urgent-care food. Fluids. Keeping him wrapped in warm towels, fresh from the dryer. Discussed pros and cons of running tests.

She cried, but agreed she didn't want us to do anything diagnostically invasive, because he was so frail. Just wanted him comfortable. Thanked me for calling.

And thank God I did call. Because when I arrived for work the next morning, Poppy was gone. Had died in the night, peacefully wrapped in his towels. I don't remember if the owner called me, or if I reached out first. Either way, I was the one who also broke the news to her. "I'm so sorry," I said. And through thick tears, she thanked me for trying, before hanging up. When she came back for her remaining dog, she was grateful we'd noticed. That we'd cared. That we'd given her the advance warning to prepare. Her Poppy hadn't died unloved.

While at least Poppy's owner had that reassurance, I prefer it if I can make a difference in the health of a pet. Sometimes I get that chance, like in the case of the dog we'll call Watson.

I had an advantage in Watson's case. Because I knew Watson's owners, and I'd met the dog several times before he was ever my patient. One of those times where the friend follows you to your place of business.

Watson had been a farm-dog, with little in the way of veterinary care in his life. They couldn't afford much more than the basics for him, but for a shepherding breed, he was pretty sweet and well-behaved. They'd taken him off the farm, and he'd go out with them on errands, day-trips, or whatever. Got a good amount of socialization once he became a town-dog.

For Christmas one year, they bought Watson one of those cheap dog-treat stockings you get from Wally World and such places. You know the ones. Nasty-looking rawhides stained red and green, twisted into a candy-cane shape. Watson must have enjoyed gnawing on it. For a while.

Over the next few days, the owners noticed their dog coughing. Gagging and hypersalivating. He would barely eat and became lethargic.

They contacted us when they couldn't take his misery anymore stating that he hadn't swallowed any of the rawhide whole but had taken his time chewing on it. They were nearly in tears for worry about their beloved pet at that point, begging me to help him. That he could keep food down, even if he wasn't excited to eat it, put an obstruction further down on our rule-out list. But the owner had an intuition about his mouth. Something was amiss there.

With Watson on the table, the veterinarian started to check him over. Everything looked within normal limits, but we saved the oral inspection for last. And when the doctor attempted to open Watson's mouth, the dog went berserk. Vocalizing, bucking, flailing, alligator-rolling, pissing, the works. Ready to bite.

The difficult truth is, because of Watson's breed, the vet made an assumption. Another poorly-behaved shepherd never taught manners. We see a lot of them, so you can't say it's not based in sound experience. A lot of shepherds get touchy about handling. Especially sensitive areas like feet, face, and ears. Mouths, certainly. What I'll say in this vet's favor, is that he's done and seen enough to know what isn't worth it. And in his wisdom, he'd decided some animals without manners aren't worth fighting. Aren't worth the risk to his or his staff's safety. Some will live and die by their own rules, and that's that.

He came to that conclusion quickly with Watson. Suggested I offer them a Band-Aid script of cough tabs to give the owners something to do, but he wasn't going to get bitten that day.

I stepped to the side with the doctor this time. Normally, I wouldn't argue much, as I'm also sick of poor behavior and fond of my digits being intact. But, as in Poppy's case, intuition was nagging me.

"This isn't right, though. That's not Watson. That's not like him to act that way. Let me get permission to sedate him and then take a closer look."

The vet was skeptical but conceded that if I really wanted to do it, fine.

I insisted.

With the worried owner's tearful permission, I restrained Watson once more while the sedative was given. The dog didn't fight us on that.

Once the drugs took effect, I carefully opened the canine's mouth. Used a flashlight to reveal the secrets of the cavity. Teeth looked fine, tongue was fine, under the tongue was fine, but … what was that? Lo and behold, there on Watson's upper palate. A wound. A red, inflamed, sore, spongy-looking wound. Almost like a burn, and about the size of a half-dollar. I didn't know if he burned his mouth somehow, had a bad reaction to that cheap Christmas rawhide, or just chewed it until the roof of his mouth was raw. Whatever the reason, it had to be immensely painful.

That wound made his outburst make sense. Watson wasn't a bad dog, he was in pain.

The vet disregarded his original script and gave the dog a blast of antibiotics and steroid. Pills to help with the soreness.

The owners struggled to afford the bill, but they were grateful to have had a reason. To know why their dog had not been himself. I had to get them to calm down in their suggestions of extra home remedy ideas, vetoing the idea of hot tea or cold drinks to soothe poor Watson's throat. ("No, don't give him anything with extreme temperatures! This isn't like your sore throat with the flu. Just the pills!")

He recovered fine and they still bring him for intermittent care to our facility. Watson might not be as thrilled to see us, but he probably didn't get the memo we helped him heal.

It helps to know your patient. It helps immensely. We may not always have that advantage, with a short window of time for a standard examination. Past SOAP records may provide some clues, but they have their limitations. At the least, a technician is an invaluable person to be an advocate for their patient.

Professionals: Tabby, or Not Tabby

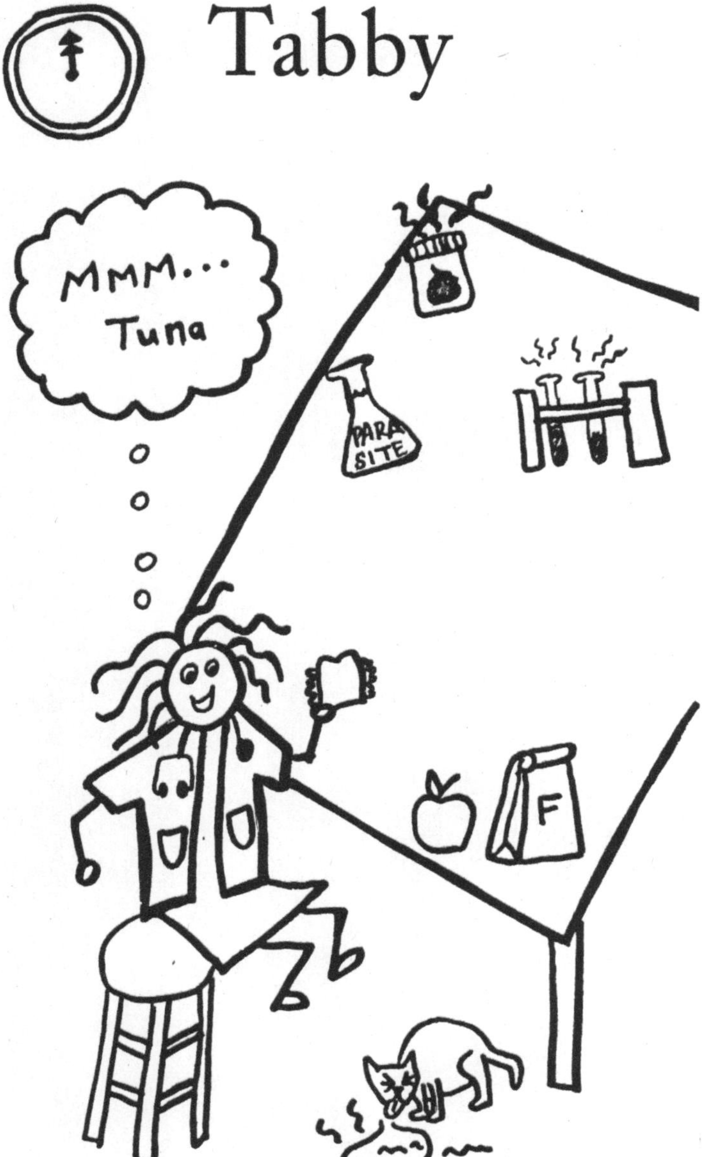

Know Thy Colleague

"I don't like that man. I must get to know him better."
—Abraham Lincoln

I hate having to get firm with a veterinarian, but sometimes that rare occasion calls for assertion on the patient's behalf.

A client called me frantically after her dachshund had been attacked by the neighbor's much bigger dog. We had a busy day, but she was a good-hearted client and I couldn't turn her away. She was someone that had had a difficult time paying off a bill in the past. We'd been patient and understanding with her then. Some time later, she'd returned and asked if she could pay it forward. We'd helped her in her time of need, and she wanted to purchase a dose of flea and tick prevention, to donate to another needy owner. At our discretion, we were allowed to select the recipient of her gift. She didn't have much, but she wanted to do her part to give back in kindness.

The veterinarian that day hadn't performed surgery in a long time. He'd injured his hand years before and had to divert all surgical procedures to the relief vet. By the time his hand healed many months later, he realized he didn't miss surgery much and was fine to let the other vet keep those cases. The occasional cat neuter, sure. No problem. But I could tell that lately, more involved procedures gave him pause. That he felt out of practice with it.

When the dachshund showed up, I was grateful that while a serious flesh wound had occurred, little Skippy wasn't critical. He was bright and alert. No major vessels or organs had been compromised. The skin was torn all the way through though, exposing the muscle layer. Certainly in need of patching up that day, but no need for hysterics.

Except I couldn't get ahold of the relief vet on her day off, and the vet that should have done it wasn't comfortable. He started to suggest that the dog might be ok to go home on antibiotics which the owner could start in a few days, as he didn't usually like to sew up such wounds the day they happened.

I was astounded.

That was the exact opposite of his typical protocols for a bite wound case. That they ought to be brought in on the *same* day, if the owner expected them to be sewn up. Otherwise, a days-old wound would just have to manage with antibiotics to help with the infection and sloughing of dead skin. (If you're wondering, yes, folks frequently bring in wounds that have already existed for several days or more.)

In Skippy's case, the owner was there the same day as the incident. As soon as she could have gotten to the clinic. Her dog was a candidate for surgical repair, and it wouldn't be terribly difficult. But the veterinarian had lost faith in himself and was clearly attempting to push her elsewhere.

I had a delicate conversation with the owner. Explaining that my surgical vet was unavailable and I could at least give her antibiotics, but I would try to triage and help her find an appointment with another clinic that could get Skippy the care he needed.

"No," was the answer I received from her. She wasn't comfortable going elsewhere, and she also had limited funds for this unexpected expense. We'd worked with her before and she hoped we would again. I had two-hundred dollars to work with.

I went back to the veterinarian's office and closed the door. Leveling with him, trying to keep my voice even and my rage under control.

"Skippy needs to have this done. She won't go anywhere else. You *know* that's not your typical recommendation, about waiting days for care. It's the opposite! Just let me sedate the dog and I'll flush out the wound myself. She's got two hundred dollars and it can cover that much, at least."

I'd made him immensely uncomfortable, but in the end, I got my stubborn way. His reluctant permission. The owner signed the sedation authorization with the understanding I was doing a very basic wound clean, staying within the budget she'd approved. No bells and whistles. Skippy would have a short road of recovering ahead. She was grateful.

I got the sweet dachshund sedated and had my VA monitor his vitals. Drugs were calculated. At the surgery table, while I was clipping up the hair around his bite wounds, the veterinarian sauntered in. Grabbed his sutures off the shelf and his other instruments from the wet pack. My bullying must have shamed him. For the first time in years, he helped me assess the wound that was his to repair, even placing a penrose drain and applying numerous sutures around the flushed laceration. Like riding a bike. The pocketed wound would drain and ooze, but it would be so much better for healing. I bit my tongue from any snide comments. Instead, gratitude took over when I found enough empathy to realize that had been a hard step back into the saddle for him, but he stepped up. He stayed through his lunch break, too, helping me to give Skippy the care he deserved.

When he later asked how much Skippy's bill was, I told him. "A hundred-and-ninety-seven dollars. I made adjustments and kept it under two hundred, as I promised her."

He held his tongue, too. It should have been more. Far more. But that was his penance and the favor she received. Except for finding the bottom of the penrose drain to be a nice chew-toy, Skippy recovered nicely.

Sometimes having to advocate so hard for my patient ensures I earn the whiskey I pour myself from my well-stocked cabinet, as was the case later that night. At least I sleep well.

And sometimes, the ethical clash just becomes too much.

It's ideal to get along with the team you work with. I do strive for that. I've been lucky enough to work with mostly amazing people over the course of my career. Alas, there was one flaw that was hard for me to overlook at a particular place of employment.

After a routine surgical procedure, the veterinarian asked me to administer the patient's post-op pain injection. No problem. Did it. Recorded it, along with the rest of the case notes.

Later in the day, that vet called me into his office.

"I noticed you made a mistake on Jackson's Rimadyl dose," he said, pointing to my notes on the computer screen. "You gave way too much. Just wanted to ask you how you came up with that number."

I was baffled and rechecked my notes. No … no, it looked right. But I'm shit at math, so I did the calculation for him once more. Still came out the same. It was correct. I told him how I'd come to that figure and his eyes narrowed quizzically.

"Well," he said. "It's … it's just not right. I'm not sure how you came up with that calculation. Jackson should be fine, but, from now on, can you just use the dosage chart posted on the cabinet?"

I agreed, because what choice did I have? But I was perplexed. I'd worked in another clinic for three years just prior and calculated the same drug nearly every day. I knew the formula from memory. Mistakes could still be made, sure, but … I hadn't made a mistake. I glanced at the chart he wanted me to refer to from then on, dismayed it wasn't all that precise. The chart entailed the use of a suggested dose tapered down to a range of weight. *Give X-amount of medication for dogs between 40—50 pounds.* That's frustrating, when I know how to calculate it more precisely for a weight of 42.8 pounds.

I stewed about it but continued with my day.

Hours later, he asked me to chat again.

"I looked up the dose officially, because it was bugging me," he admitted. "And it turns out, you're right. I'm not sure why our chart's off, but your calculation is what's recommended on the Rimadyl label."

No shit, was what I wanted to say, but I elected for something less provocative.

"Oh, ok, great."

"So … it's more than what we usually give to patients, so I guess we'll have to refigure our prices on the surgery estimates from now on. To cover that cost."

"Sure," I agreed.

So, I calmed down and was content. Glad to have my small victory. Vet acknowledged his mistake and said we'd make it right. And more important than my ego, we'd prevent dogs from being underdosed on pain medication from then on.

Until we didn't.

It lasted no more than two weeks. The lucky dogs in that short window got their proper dosing, but after that, the vet changed his mind once more. As he explained to me, his clients watched budgets closely, and they were sure to notice the price increase from one year to the next. The idea of confrontation made him uncomfortable, so we were going to go back to the original dosing chart.

Ahem. You might be wondering how much cheddar is on the table. The price jump in question was probably ten or fifteen bucks, at most. To administer the full amount of medication that ought to have been given, per patient. We're not talking about breaking the average person's bank, here. For ten dollars more, we can lessen potential pain your pet might be experiencing. Isn't that what you trust us to do, when we perform surgical procedures on your animal? To do so as painlessly as possible? Seems ethical to me, but what the fuck do I know?

He wasn't wrong about the culture of his client base. I saw for myself they watched prices closely, and, as he said, some would surely notice the small spike. But where I found him to be unjustifiably wrong, was that he couldn't even bear the thought of just a quick explanation. To even try. Certain it would be a failed conversation.

"Hey, so the cost of the drugs has increased a little bit more than it was last year, but it's very effective at keeping Roo's pain under control."

Was that so hard? If someone asked, it's really all that needed to be said. I'd sure as fuck like my dog to wake up from anesthesia without being in pain.

I learned to be a tech in a culture where, if you believed in the value of your service, you promoted it. Sure, we inevitably encounter a certain percentage who can't afford it, even if they have confidence in us. But that has to be present first. Fucking confidence. To know what we offer for our patients and their families, and to follow that mission firmly. When a situation is beyond our expertise, we refer it to the expert we think can help. Until then, we owe it to our patients to extend the best quality of care we're able to provide.

I moved on from that employment, to find a clinic culture I could get behind.

Emotionally Charged

"Dogs have given us their absolute all. We are the center of their universe. We are the focus of their love and faith and trust. They serve us in return for scraps. It is without a doubt the best deal man has ever made."
—Roger A. Caras

Service animals versus emotional support animals. Let's get this over with.

If you don't know the difference, a service animal is a dog that has gone through a rigorous training process and has been properly certified to assist a human in need, with a specific disability. Such canines are recognized by the ADA. Canines are the only allowable species for a service animal. And yeah. They're expensive, due to their skill. Well into the thousands of dollars.

An emotional support animal (ESA), in contrast, does not have to go through any training whatsoever. You can claim any species as your support. You want an emotional support chicken? Bearded dragon? Alpaca? Whatever. Go for it. *You* (Homo sapiens) are the criteria for an emotional support animal, not the other way around. Any human who can claim a mental health disorder has grounds for keeping an ESA. They are not recognized as service animals, though.

Let me say upfront: I am completely in favor of people having animals for emotional support. Mental health deserves awareness and respect, alongside physical health. It's been well documented in scientific studies that animals can provide stress relief for their humans by decreasing cortisol and increasing oxytocin. The power of a bonding relationship. In short, animals have the capability to be incredibly healing.

Just like those benefiting from a service animal, I truly, one thousand percent, believe there are people who deserve an emotional support animal. Folks with mental health struggles whose lives are enhanced due to the companionship of their pet. Those who have a right to the certificate, obtainable by their doctor or therapist.

There's always a "but."

But what gets my goat? No shocker, as I'm not unique to making this argument, is the abuse, overuse, and mishandling of the system. ESA certifications and the marked vests for the animals to wear are entirely too easy to obtain. Criteria for an ESA stretched to include basically anyone, if you're willing to say you could use one. "I enjoy petting my dog," seems to be all it takes.

For a while, I got an influx of calls at the clinic. People asking if we, the veterinary staff, could assist them in getting their pet ESA-certified. I was baffled at first and then double-checked to make sure I wasn't outdated on my information. Nope. After that, I'd have to explain to the callers that it had nothing to do with the veterinary team. Nil. Zero. Zip. Why? Because other than providing healthcare services for your animal, (which we *do* recommend) there's nothing about an ESA requiring training. Even if said creature did come trained, we vet folks wouldn't be the ones qualified to judge it. No; what they needed, as I tried to gently explain to those inquiring, was a note from their human doctor, therapist, or psychiatrist authorizing their ESA requirement.

If you're wondering why I claim abuse of the system, it's because we see it frequently. It's not hard to find a scam certificate online for a small fee. A vest doesn't prove anything, either. Anybody can buy a vest. Animals come into my office wearing vests emblazoned with both titles. ESA ones, quite commonly. One couple has put it on every single one of their (numerous) pets. *Service Animal* has even been seen on a few that definitely don't qualify, and it's fucking insulting to those who need it. I shouldn't see that *Service Animal* vest nearly as often as I have.

One big impetus for people doing this is for living arrangements. Usually, rental properties. When a landlord doesn't want to allow pets, it's an easy excuse to work around the rule. It's harder for the landlord to say 'no' to the tenant's pet if they claim it's a service animal or an ESA. We see and hear the suggestion thrown out with ease. "Just say it's an ESA, and then you can have Tinkles live with you!"

In some cases, it's even the rental staff who are the accountable party.

I've got an old pal since elementary school days, who is a rule-follower. Her whole life. Kindhearted, straight A student in school, ambitious, hated getting into trouble, by-the-book, type-A personality. Yeah, not at all like me. Getting her to drop the F-bomb for the first time in high school was a major cause for celebration among our sophomoric little gaggle of friends.

I swear, we do have some things in common that warrant our friendship. But I digress. She's a good person. A morally conscious person.

She and her husband lived in a major city, in a nice apartment building. On a recent visit back "home," we met up. Somehow this topic arose. Someone asked my opinion, or maybe I just rudely decided to subject them to it. As I was ranting about the rental scenario, she interrupted me.

Old friend was one of those people, certifying her dog as an emotional support so she could be allowed to live with them in their apartment complex. I was stunned, but more so when she told me why. It was due to the instigating push from the apartment's *own* staff. While it was advertised as a dog-friendly establishment, there was an unexpected weight limit on pets. Their dog surpassed that boundary line.

Though frustrated, she prepared herself to face a continuing apartment search elsewhere. Until the staff surprised her with a whispered hint. Like an under-the-table transaction. *Nudge, nudge. Wink, wink. Hey, just register Susie-Q as an ESA …*

If they were telling her how to bend their own establishment rule, then what was the point? Given her personality, this old friend was still conflicted as to whether to go through with it. After clinical assessment, family discussions, advice, and carefully reviewing the vague definitions of a broken system, they agreed that indeed, she met those foundational requirements. Nothing dishonest. When telling me about the scenario, she acknowledged it was a flimsy and disappointing premise. Nonetheless, in need of housing, they moved forward with the rental apartment. Susie-Q gained clearance to be her ESA.

It's not her fault the system is flawed. That she was asked to participate in the ethically ambiguous loophole. I can't help but think it would be better if the rental property had adjusted their allowance for pets instead. That would be a greater favor to actual service or emotional support animals, than encouraging a rule-bending frame of mind.

Besides rental perks, the bigger issue comes about in public. Those citizens who want to be able to take their animal anywhere, with carte blanche permission. Grocery store, airport, library, wherever. I'm sure everyone's run into a questionable guest in public. It's a delicate thing for business owners to question, which is why customers get away with breaking rules when only service animals are meant to be allowed. Often, animals that are untrained, terribly behaved, or aggressive are the ones strolling around. One of my vet buddies would text me from her weekly grocery trip after getting an eyeful of an unfortunate specimen perusing the produce aisle nearby. Intact, flea-bitten, filthy *Service* vest askew, and tugging on his retractable leash out of eagerness to put his signature claim on the corn cob racks …

Piss on corn isn't the end of the world, no. But there are horror stories out there about such violators. Animals causing bodily injuries in public. Fake service animals have been observed intimidating real service animals, making it difficult for them to perform their duties. You can use your imagination.

It gives a bad name to the legitimate ones. Undermining their authenticity and then causing suspicion for the folks who do need them.

I'm pleading with humanity to help improve and protect our standards. One of the greatest marks of civility is how we take care of each other. There are those who need and deserve to have the service or emotional companion animal in public situations. If you're not in one of those categories, stop taking advantage. Stop corrupting the rules to be pointless. Stop eroding the worthiness of true cases. It's a massive disservice to your fellow humans and to the animals with jobs to perform. Don't be the reason we can't have nice things. Fucking hell. Now, someone help me down off this SOAPBOX. I hate heights.

Drop It: Anthropomorphism in Veterinary Culture

"The ones who have a voice must speak for those who are voiceless."
—Oscar Romero

The following is modified, but I've tried submitting it to professional veterinary publications, as a stand-alone article. It came about, oh, some-whereabouts after finishing a secondary degree, while still rolling over thoughts in my head about formal study of animal behavior, various animal-related -ologies, a bit of ecology, as well as research into the convoluted world of animal rights versus welfare arguments. Greatly influenced by these and a book called *Nature Wars* by Jim Sterba, as well as some points by Marian Stamp Dawkins from *Why Animals Matter*, it was all fascinating stuff. I wondered how it applied to my veterinary context. I'm not a brilliant researcher, but I started to worry about some of the disconnects in front of me. Eventually, this … thing formed out of the troubled musings.

It's a plea to the veterinary community about their language. About awareness of what they know and what they don't know. Only received crickets in return, by the way. I'm not surprised by the rejection from those publishers. Because, frankly, the would-be article trashed some of the current trends in vet culture and surely stepped on some toes. Nonetheless, here it is.

You're welcome.

—

I swore I would never be one of those owners dressing my dog in cutesy sweaters and bows. When I heard references to *fur babies*, *pet parents*, *four-legged children*, or other such terms that humanized our animal companions, I cringed. During my early years of experience in a clinic, I would see those bedazzled patients and inwardly roll my eyes, while outwardly gushing to appease the client.

And now, as I write this, my miniature rat terrier snoozes next to me on the recliner, while I peruse browser tabs online, shopping for dog sweaters. The adorable woodsy one with a moose, prominently featured. I promise myself, it's *only* because it's winter and I live in the Midwest. Ooh, what about the classic Christmas sweater, or the conversion Velcro-jacket? She's been hanging out next to the heater the last three days, I remind myself, as I submit payment for the items in my online shopping cart. She needs it. She's only nine pounds.

Still, that utilitarian necessity is encroaching frivolity. Hypocrite? Absolutely. I'm working on it.

The veterinary market has grown rapidly in recent decades, and the expectations of consumers have grown with it. Overall, it ought to be a positive trend. That is why we're here. To improve the lives of animals under our stewardship—companion, livestock, research, or zoo. To strengthen the human-animal bond. To educate our clients on how they can achieve healthier choices for their animals. If one needs selfish motivation (for those less fond of, or uninterested in animals), it's been proven that quality care of fauna, in turn, comes back to serve human interest. No one who's made a career in the veterinary world would say otherwise.

It is because I've dedicated my professional career to improving quality of life for animals that I make the undoubtedly unpopular assertion: anthropomorphizing the creatures we love so much undermines our very own mission.

Anthropomorphism is the act of attributing human qualities to non-humans. Take Donald Duck, for example. A talking duck that wears a sailor shirt and hat. Or most Disney animal characters.

I'm far from the first to talk about this problematic concept. And don't forget, I'm just as guilty as the next person, buying those dog sweaters. But I want to be better. That's the whole point of why I go to work every day—to help animals.

Who cares? Why then, is anthropomorphizing animals such a big deal? What do our word choices matter? What's wrong with *fur baby*?

First, let's touch on the disconnect from nature. Applying language that relates an animal to a human-form will ultimately be a disservice to that animal, and to us. They may live in our homes, they may be distant descendants of wilder ancestors, and they may have adapted to a cushy lifestyle with regular dinner service, but our society needs to bear in mind their dog, cat, or chinchilla are entirely that—a different species. As more of the world's population has moved to city or suburb-dwelling communities, our human bond with nature has dwindled. That doesn't help matters. Fewer of us live among "the wild," nor must we work so hard for necessities. Our own ancestors understood better their relationship to land and nature. Nowadays, when we interact with those areas, we need signage to tell us what should be common sense. *Don't feed bears. Don't approach bison. Beware of night bandits; secure your trash!*

(You think I wouldn't love to feed a raccoon, too? Of course I fucking would. My dumb ass knows better, but I'd still *want* to. There. Hypocrite again.)

Commonplace anthropomorphism promotes such dangerous behavior. Encourages us to think of wildlife as cuddly and approachable. It's a blatant disregard for biology.

Modern conveniences, designed to create easier lives for us every day, make for a divide between humans and the natural world. Under this massive umbrella includes the increasing popularity of pet products on the market and services available to consumers. Some practical, sure. Some are ...not. Dog poop tent or cat bum-hole cover, anyone? With these trends, I wonder about the consequences. As far as animal ownership is concerned, I've read reports about Millennials and Gen-Zers being more 'obsessed' with their pets than their parents, or grandparents before them. I'm betting that pattern continues. The more we 'baby' our pets, the more likely we are to put that same assumption of cuddliness onto actual wildlife. Spoiler alert: it nearly always has catastrophic results for the natural world.

It isn't really a veterinary team's place to remark on wildlife, unless they've had a specialty interest. However, it is interesting we're expected to have expertise in an area for which we've had very little education. Numerous veterinary clients have called to ask if we can give insight about a problem on their land with a pest, or if we could look at the wounded critter they encountered on their morning walk. For the latter, I've had to redirect them to a refuge that is qualified for such handling, or simply to recommend leaving said creature alone.

I've never forgotten one of our top clients rushing into the lobby one morning, making a beeline for me behind the desk and uttering the most bone-chilling "Help me! *Help* me!"

Before any inquiries could escape my mouth, he'd pushed a fledgling bird into my hand that had fallen from its nest. At once, a cascade of bird mites crawled down from their host to cover my thumb and wrist. So thick, it looked as if I'd pulled on a glove. The bird was lucky I (barely) squashed the knee-jerk reaction of flinging him and his parasitic pals across the room. We offered food and kept the bird for a brief few hours of observation so the client would feel better but then released it back to nature. As I said, my facility didn't have the ability or the license for treating it.

Most veterinarians and technicians don't have to take courses in wildlife biology, ecology, conservation, and the like to achieve their credentials. Purely because I was a nerd who dipped my toes into some of those areas, there were those eye-opener accounts that quickly made me realize I didn't know as much as I thought I did about natural history. And this was after I'd obtained my RVT license. We could use a humbling reminder to preach what we know about medicine, but stay in our lane when we don't know about the great outdoors.

The buildup of all that was to say this: Devaluation is what's at stake.

I've always had a passion for animals. I like 'em better than most people. I admit it. On the rare occasion I'm invited to a party, you'll probably find me along a wall trying to befriend the host's dog. Other veterinary professionals might say the same. Regardless of my opinion of fellow humans, I do recognize the value of human life. Obviously, I place value on animal life, too. Without getting into religious beliefs or physiological and psychological makeup—these two things are not the same. We are sentient beings, both. Deserving of respect and understanding. We are *connected*, but not equivalent.

It's become my increasing concern that the upward trend of treating ourselves as *pet parents* is contributing to disrespect for humans. I'm not a parent myself, so I can't speak from experience in this regard, but I do know many parents are offended by the notion of daring to compare raising animals to raising children. Thus, my beef with anthropomorphism.

Consider the insane mob mentality that comes from social media exploiting abuse cases in the news. Everyone's seen them. That disgruntled individual trying to slander the reputation of a business or individual. Angry clients spewing online about a vet clinic, boarding facility, or a professional, followed by the uproar from folks anywhere in the world. Threats of professional shunning, cancellation, violence, or even death ensue. All because of an assumption about a situation that, frankly, they probably know little about, from an already one-sided version.

I want to pull for my vet community. People who spent time, money, and energy to do what they do. They care. They care every day, even if they're burnt out from caring. I'm not saying we shouldn't be held accountable for poor quality work when it does happen. Medicine *should* have a certain amount of regulative oversight. And we do. Inside any clinic, there's a chain of command. Outside, we all answer to regulating boards that issue our licenses, set legal practice standards, inspect our premises, and review significant case conflicts. Still, at the end of the day, we want to remember those professionals are humans of value and worth. Not someone who should be 'cancelled' (I despise this fucking term) by keyboard warriors or threatened with real violent action, because someone got second- or third- or nineteenth-hand information about what happened to someone else's animal.

Stop encouraging your client to think of their pet as their *furry child.* Anthropomorphic terms reinforce the skewed comparison. We're promoting demeaning behavior toward ourselves as a roundabout result. In a field that seeks continued growth but is hurting for help. Feeling undervalued, degraded, and burnt out from emotionally demanding situations are among the top reasons it's hard to retain good help.

Our clients look to us for guidance in so many aspects about the life, health, and even death of their pets. We ask them to put their trust in our expertise. And if we're to do our job properly, the veterinary team owes it to them to live up to a higher standard. That includes the language we use when we educate.

What about the preposterous notion of interspecies consent? With vets needing consent from animal patients to perform their job? Last point, I promise.

If you ever read Rudyard Kipling's *The Jungle Book*, you might recall his characters (animals with the capacity for complex thought—sound familiar?) discussing the Law of Man versus the Law of the Jungle. Kipling gives far more credit to the nature of animals than to their counterparts. But as he establishes, the rules by which we govern ourselves are not the same across species. As the man-character (Mowgli) is becoming educated in the dominion of human masters over their elephants, for example, he questions the use of the *ankus*, which is the sharp tool utilized by the elephant handler to control the animal, usually as a form of punishment (regarded these days as a cruel instrument, and rightly so). When Mowgli asks the wise panther Bagheera why an ankus is being used by thrusting it into an elephant's head, Bagheera answers him: "To teach them Man's Law …"

Take the fictionalized classic story with a grain of salt. But can anyone who has ever studied animal behavior, Darwin's theory of natural selection, or even seen an episode of *Planet Earth* deny animals operate by their own rules and instincts? Those Laws of the Jungle have little to do with human will. And while many a good dog will seek to please their owner, they don't have the same understanding of our human motives as we do.

So. Why are we asking for consent from animals, with this new popular wave of initiatives? Veterinary folks will know the program I'm talking about, intended to eliminate fear.

Don't get me wrong, y'all. There are definite pros. I support a better emotional experience for our patients. I want to applaud every effort to understand the species in our care. Utilizing calming pheromones, proper analgesics to reduce pain, sedation where necessary, or creating an environment without overload of stressful stimuli? All good things. A refresher on those strategies can be a great thing.

For however many thousands of animals I've seen in practice, though, I can only make an interpretation of what their body language is telling me. I like to think I'm more often correct than not, but it is still that. An interpretation. They don't use the same language as me. Watch for physical cues and make it the most positive experience possible? Definitely.

If a patient arrives frightened, aggressive, or in pain, the last thing we want is to make the situation worse for them. We owe them good care. Alas, I've heard this program's objectives discussed in an irrational way by its promoters. Expecting a cat to dutifully place a paw in my hand and "ask" me to trim its nails, or kitty goes home without the trim? I'm sorry, we're bordering on the absurd. At a veterinary conference I attended, the program's concept was introduced to a room full of shocked professionals with this very example.

I think there's a good balance to be found, because, simply, significant good exists in this newer movement. However, an animal cannot sign off on its consent in a language we can accept in a court of human law. Hello, anthropomorphism. That silly interspecies issue.

For those wondering what could be in the cons column, other critics of the movement feel that it's an unnecessary marketing cash grab. To acquire a feel-good label that appeals to clients. Offering training on topics that credentialed veterinary staff are already educated in. Some call it a gimmick, too, with an insulting implication that if clinics don't pay pricey fees for the program's certification, they must have no regard for the animals. For me, there's a sense of elitism as a business model. If clients understand they're investing in behavioral exercises that may require multiple vet visits, go for it, but for standard vet practice? I can't imagine telling most clients, who'd be pissed about the inconvenience to their time (and precious money), that we didn't perform the medical service because Boomer didn't feel like having his nails cut.

Anyway. Pros, cons, and forever trying to find the right balance. I'm a sucker for balance and moderation.

If you're an animal activist wanting to fight for the rights of animals, or even good welfare of your veterinary patients, don't do your mission a disservice by humanizing that animal. Those opposed to your intentions will find you far less credible when you use emotional or anthropomorphic arguments. They need to see factual, data-driven reasoning.

For my purposes? Our patients are sentient and deserving of respect but cannot be proven capable of understanding human day-to-day motives in a clinical setting. Frankly, I'm going to see a lot of patients not getting the care they need, if I'm waiting for their anthropomorphic permission. Besides, I want to promote proper respect for both human and animal. To honor our connectedness in a better fashion.

I am a veterinary technician because I wanted to be a voice for voiceless animals. That's my job, in a nutshell. Improving their existence. Enhancing the co-existence between our species and theirs. But that doesn't mean forcing a human agenda on them. The 'Law of Man' makes no sense to an animal. Let's remember the difference between speaking their language and being their voice. And let's try to remove some of those dog Halloween costumes from our shopping cart.

For the Sake of Levity: Anal Gland Espressos

Anal gland expression. It's another hard phrase for clients to wrap their brains around, apparently. I mean, for me it seems pretty straightforward, but I'm the lucky winner who gets to perform the task multiple times a day. Dogs (and cats) have anal glands. Anal glands have to be expressed when they can't do it on their own. Anal gland expression.

Thank God humans don't have them.

Clients don't like to talk about it. I had one lady, perturbed by her scooting dog. I began to explain what it was that we needed to check. Didn't get far. She shut me down as soon as she heard something called an 'anal gland' existed, saying she didn't want to know. Just, no. Absolutely not.

I had to kindly say, "Well, Rufus still needs to have *it* done, because it's uncomfortable and can cause a prob—"

"Fine, take him in the back and just do it. But I won't hear about it. Ugh."

One of those squeamish procedures with a foul odor. If you get even the tiniest speck of that liquid on you, you're doing laundry, or no one is going to want to be in the same room as you the rest of the day. We've all had that moment, after thinking you've properly cleaned the exam room, yet the stench hasn't left your nostrils, so you ask one of your trusty coworkers to do the sniff test on you, trying to locate it. And yes, sometimes we've celebrated when the olfactorily-offensive liquid shoots across the room. We revert into prepubescent boys, proud of the height it reached or the expansiveness of the spray across the wall.

We celebrate far less when it's hit us in the face, or God forbid, the mouth. Yeah, it's happened. Not to me, thank fuck, but I've heard the horror stories. If you know what's good for you, don't talk while you're expressing one of those glands.

Those clients that can bear to know of the existence of the anatomy still can't help being hilarious when they request "it" to be done. We hear endless variations of 'the tushy thing.' For those that really struggle, I suggest they keep it simple. "If you can't remember it, just tell us Snuggles needs his bum squeezed. We'll know what you mean."

One of my regular clients quite obviously had a crush on the veterinarian. She watched while he performed the necessary process on her pug, and couldn't help but comment, "Ooh, he could squeeze my butt that way."

That should make you cringe hard enough to crumple into yourself. Nice lady, I swear. But yikes. Moving on.

Hands down, the best I've heard is the client request for "a butt extraction."

Just think about that one.

And since we're talking about putting appendages in animal backsides, I think there's an immature crowd that always wants to know if veterinary professionals have put their arm inside a cow, so I'll stick this here. In my case, with my limited large animal know-how, the answer is yes. But only once, in tech school. We were offered the opportunity to practice a pregcheck during bovine rotation, and I took a turn. Nervously administering the full-sleeve plastic glove with a healthy dollop of lubrication. My fellow classmates and I happened to be a group with mostly small animal experience between us. None of us country girls, like others in the class. So, there we were, giggling at the absurdity of the new experience. When it was time, the others hesitated, so I volunteered to go first.

The older veteran veterinarian dryly informed me how to approach, and what I was palpating for, in the rectal exam. My fingers felt along the different surfaces, and I knew I was in over my head—figuratively—as I had no idea how to discern one part from the next. It all felt the same to a newbie. Partway, I gasped, shocked at the sudden sensation of my arm getting pulled inside further. Buried nearly to my shoulder. Somewhere exists a photo of this moment, taken by a classmate. Incredulous humor written all over my face.

"Ah, yeah, you'll reach about that far and feel suction," the vet instructor added, noting my expression. He'd done it so many times in his career, he was surely marveling at the lack of large-animal smarts between the students assigned to him.

Eventually, I finished my turn and watched the other girls, one by one, as we continued moving cows through the chute. Appreciating them all going through the same experience, but none so much as the last girl. Like me, she gasped when the sensation of suction pulled her in further.

"Oh, it's giving me a hug!" she exclaimed, grinning from ear-to-ear.

The veterinarian's face fell into his palm in disbelief.

Pandemic

"COVID-19 is the result of being infected with severe acute respiratory syndrome coronavirus 2 (or SARS-CoV-2). In addition to humans, some non-human animals may become infected with SARS-CoV-2. However, there is no compelling evidence that domestic animals readily transmit SARS-CoV-2 to people under normal circumstances."
—AVMA

Waiting to board a return flight to the U.S. from Scotland, I scrolled through my phone out of boredom. With the feed refreshed a few times, social media had worn out its welcome. Email spam had been deleted. Figured I ought to check the news of the world next. Alas, there wasn't much of interest in the top headlines for me.

It was January of 2020. My husband had bought me surprise tickets for my birthday earlier in 2019, and we'd just enjoyed an amazing New Year's trip to the Scottish Highlands. Bar hopping and enjoying picturesque fireworks over the Caledonian Canal of Inverness on Hogmanay seemed a good starting omen for the year. Followed by numerous other beautiful sights and experiences. Little did we know we'd gotten a last vacation in the nick of time. There wouldn't be another for quite a while.

Headlines may have bored me, but I was always more intrigued by the weird or obscure news. I had nothing else to do in that airport, so I scrolled all the way to the bottom of the webpage looking for anything that might kill a few minutes. Lo and behold, there was a word that caught my attention. I clicked on the link and skimmed through the brief report.

"Anything interesting?" my husband inquired, rejoining me with a coffee he'd purchased from a kiosk.

"There's a coronavirus outbreak," I answered. "In some small village in China. All kinds of businesses getting shut down, looks like. And they're closing the borders."

"Huh," he said noncommittally.

And that was it, the first time in January we heard of the coronavirus. The one about to cripple our world as we knew it. A bottom-of-the-barrel news story about some faraway place with their inconvenient troubles. It had mainly piqued my curiosity because I vaccinate canines against their *own* strain of coronavirus every day in practice. And for morbid fascination, I'd taken just enough microbiology and viewed or read thrillers about viral outbreaks. Stories like *The Hot Zone* (by Richard Preston) or *Contagion.* Honestly, I knew little to nothing about a human strain of coronavirus, though. Nor did I expect it to affect me.

We made it back home to the States safe and sound. I may have mentioned the news story to a coworker once, but mostly forgot about it, until weeks later, when it began picking up traction. I started to become slightly concerned seeing the virus had spread out of Wuhan. Folks were beginning to take health precautions in other areas.

At the end of the month, we received the tragic news that my husband's stepfather had passed away suddenly. After talks with my in-laws about arrangements, plans were made for my husband and I to make a trip down South for a few days to be with his mother.

Just a few weeks before, I'd have thought nothing of a quick continental flight. Now, in early February, the headlines were becoming louder. I was concerned. Working in a medical facility, I had easy access to surgical face masks. I borrowed two for the trip, packing them carefully in my carry-on bag. When we arrived at the airport, I pulled mine out of my bag and hooked the straps around my ears. Pinched the nosepiece to fit to my face, before the parking shuttle bus picked us up. I offered the second to my husband.

He rolled his eyes at me and declined. "You're really gonna wear that?"

I insisted. I wore it the whole time in the airports and on our two flights until we arrived, only pulling it aside to briefly eat or drink. My husband wasn't the only one to find me strange. I got a lot of weird looks for wearing a mask on February 6, 2020. Just to prove to my teasing spouse he couldn't unnerve me, I even posted my picture wearing it. "Travel couture. Get away from me," I captioned it. I didn't wear it for the duration of visiting family, but when it was time for our return flight, once again, I donned the mask. My husband's unused one.

By late February, I was definitely concerned. I don't remember when it started becoming headline news for the U.S., but I know I wasn't alone by then. Certainly by March, everyone was aware of it. Footage of the spread throughout Europe, and especially Italy, alarmed and saddened me. If it could happen there, it would certainly happen in America, too. Our world was too inter-connected. It was just going to be a matter of time. Husband, who had previously thought it was all fuss that would die down to nothing, came around, too. We were on the same page.

I'm sure most can recall the confusion and disorganization of March of 2020. Safety protocols were up for consideration in the Midwest, but most places, not yet fully fleshed out, and barely enforced. We were all still pronouncing the title of the virus with care—COVID-19.

—

In the veterinary office, we had a few trickling phone calls from owners starting to be concerned about the effect on their pets. We only had snippets of information, the same as everyone else. By March 13, I was able to share a post on my clinic's social media page from the AVMA (American Veterinary Medical Association), stating that there were no known cases in domestic animals.

Husband and I attended our town's St. Paddy's Day pub crawl later that weekend. But already, something felt uncomfortable about it. Here, we'd seen shocking footage of coronavirus cases shutting down other countries. Devastatingly high numbers of deaths in a short period of time, and no politely manageable way for some of them to deal with such a volume. Travel restrictions. Closed public spaces. The beginnings of social distancing. Calls for everything to be cancelled. Suddenly, hopping from bar to bar for festive green beer felt ridiculous. The crowd of people around me, intimidatingly unnecessary. Foolish. I looked at my husband and requested we go home from the event early. He didn't argue with me.

The following Monday, my veterinary clinic had our first serious sit-down about what was happening in the outside world. By then, everyone had to acknowledge this was a big deal. The AVMA was beginning to address veterinary facilities with their recommendations, too. When your accrediting organization makes a statement, you're compelled to listen. You can disobey, but that's certainly going to be frowned upon and likely lead to other consequences. It was time to think about where the veterinary field sat in the grand scheme of things. And while fields of animal medicine and research are filled with professionals who understand the importance of our patients and subjects, we had to swallow a hard truth. People come first.

We were still deemed a crucial business for in-person operation. Not in the category that could be expected to work from home. No. I still drove to work every day in the overall quieter streets. Still, measures needed to be taken.

First, we were asked to streamline our appointments. Discourage unnecessary family members from attending. We made a policy that only one person could bring the pet into the appointment. Social distancing was attempted inside the clinic. *Stand behind this line, don't lean over the counter leering at the receptionist, or hang too close to your coworker if you don't have to.* Like anywhere else, clients who felt unwell were asked to cancel or reschedule.

Soon, the types of appointments were up for discussion. Discontinuing unnecessary or non-urgent visits was strongly encouraged by the veterinary board. It was up to the individual clinics to determine the particulars, so we had to have some group discussions surrounding the chopping block. Nail trims? Nope! (Ok, we might have been gleeful about that one.) Annual vaccines for an older pet that had already been well-vaccinated? Postpone. Grooming services? Cut entirely, for the time being. We didn't know yet for how long. A week? Two weeks? A month? Six? Longer …?

The grooming appointments were an initial point of contention. Our groomer, to be fair, didn't rely heavily on the paycheck and could get by comfortably enough without it. With that reassurance, it seemed an obvious first thing that should go. The manager and I agreed on that, as did the relief vet (Dr. Y). Haircuts were not something we were going to risk our health and safety over. Not worth it. It would be a ludicrous thing to maintain. This was near the beginning of everything, and we were scared.

The manager went to clear that decision with the vet that owned the practice (Dr. X), and apparently, Dr. X was dismissive. Citing it was no big deal to continue groom appointments, so we'd be keeping them. I was livid when I heard. It was the help staff that handled those appointments. Manager, receptionist, assistant, tech, or the groomer herself. The face-to-face hand-offs from owner to staff member. Whoever happened to be manning the front desk when an owner walked in the door. *We* were the ones at first risk in that scenario. Not the vets.

My manager is a kind person and handles a lot of shit I could never bring myself to deal with all the time. Billing, tracking down clients who owe, inventory and pricing, scheduling. She's not a confrontational person, and I know she tends to shy away from it. I'm the consummate introvert, myself, and could never claim I enjoy the clash, either. Yet, I'll do it if I must. When my temper simmered down, I knew I had to speak for myself and the others. To my benefit, I worked in a place where I had a voice and leverage. It was a small clinic, and Dr. X needed me. Which is not something I try to take unfair advantage of, but if I want to put my foot down about an issue, I have grounds to be heard. So, I went to Dr. X's office, and while I didn't know if my voice was as steady as I would have liked, I made myself clear.

"If we're doing grooming appointments still, I don't want to work."

Dr. X paused from writing at his desk and looked at me. No angry reply, no scolding lecture. To his credit, he mulled over that realization. As the horrid cliché went, these were uncertain times. He was going to have to be considerate of his staff's concerns about this whole virus business and take it seriously. Dr. X conceded, and that was that. Grooming was cut off, for the time being.

Dr. X came up with a suggestion of his own, shortly after. Reading through CDC guidelines, he pointed out that we should eliminate wearing our wristwatches. Another potential fomite that could harbor germs. As I was the ringleader for implementing clinic safety protocols, he was looking directly at me when he said it. After getting my way about the grooming appointments, it was a concession I was all too happy to make. He may have been getting into the spirit of the issues or wanting to exert his own authoritative measure. Whatever. It served my goals, so I obligingly took my watch off and left it at home from then on. Added the note for the staff guidelines. No watches should be worn. We'd use wall clocks from then on to measure heart rates and such.

One of the bigger concerns was supplies. Everywhere in the world, not just in the veterinary industry. Personal protective equipment (PPE) and surgical supplies were in high demand, and not enough were available to keep up. With human medical fields becoming more desperate, the AVMA called upon veterinarians to do their part. Elective surgeries needed to be postponed, too. IV fluids might need to be donated. If we had surgical gloves to spare, they may be more greatly needed by human doctors. Even non-sterile gloves for other procedures. Surgical drapes used in our veterinary surgery were considered a means to fashion N95 mask coverings for human medical staff, so they could preserve the longevity of their equipment.

We set aside a small stock of these items for our own emergency use, but the rest were piled up, in case they should be requested. The hospital in my town ended up asking for donations for the N95 mask covers, among other things. They gave their specifications on the dimensions. I cut down sixty-four pieces of our clinic's surgical drape for human healthcare workers.

By March 18, our vet clinic posted our expected list of client protocols to be followed, via in-clinic signage and on our media pages. It was a trying first few days getting it all figured out. Herding clients around the building was a nightmare. No one stood where they were supposed to. Few people yet had awareness of courteous posture. Some rude folks thought it was funny to fake-cough on the receptionist. Sanitizing everything clients touched was becoming increasingly hard to keep up with, in between every appointment. No flow to the process. And I'll say it; my clients are notoriously bad about showing up early for appointments. Sometimes as early as forty-five minutes. If that describes you? Please stop. We've told you to come when we want you there. You stress us out by being so early. It's not politely punctual. It's rude and disrespectful of our time. Anyways. The sanitizing. My hands were raw from handling so much disinfectant at a higher virucidal rate of dilution, plus the increased handwashing. It wasn't going to be long before they were cracked and bleeding.

By the 23rd, we had a more firm posting for our clinic. Curbside service was mandatory.

Yet another drastic change for us to navigate. It took time. Many hiccups. Euthanasia appointments were the only exception to allowing in a masked client, two at most, to be with their pet in its final moments. Careful monitoring to make sure everything they touched was sanitized afterward. Otherwise, we figured out the flow of curbside service, and it worked well for us. When a client arrived at their appointed time, they either called our lobby phone from the safety of their vehicle, or knocked on the door to alert us. A masked staff member would run outside to fetch the animal. Or the same process for picking up a prescription. Items were delivered out to the parking lot. Discussions were had outside from a safe social distance. Or over the phone if the weather was less than ideal. Bills were paid over the phone, or cards carried inside on behalf of the client, then sanitized and returned. It wasn't worth the trouble of having signatures on receipts.

I had to laugh at some of the early exchanges. I went to grab a lady's pet, seeing her mask up the whole time she sat alone in her car and as I grabbed the carrier from her. But when she wanted to speak to me, her face not more than two feet from mine, she pulled her mask down to her chin. Gabbed away. Missing the point entirely.

Some didn't mind curbside service, content to sit in their car and wait. Catching up on work, scrolling through their phones, or reading a book to pass the time. One even complained they wanted more waiting time, when I returned their pet sooner than expected. For many clients, though, it took months to get on board. They couldn't bear the thought of having to send their precious pet into the clinic without them present. Separation anxiety was rampant, and not necessarily by the pets.

I'll be honest. It was a hard thing to be sympathetic over. I get people want what's best for their pet. So do we. Duh. Kind of why we're here. It's another one of those things folks don't realize is insulting when they break down about letting us borrow their animal for five or ten minutes. We don't exist to traumatize animals unnecessarily.

At the same time, businesses that decided their workers could do their jobs from home were making the leap. A curfew wasn't mandated in our town, but it might as well have, for how deserted public areas became. Large social gatherings were kiboshed. Only necessary errands were looked upon kindly, and the hope was that you loaded up and did your shopping efficiently. No time for idle browsing. Social distancing was expected.

Shamefully, I used to think up excuses to run into Walgreens on my way home. Just to have some other place I could go besides work and home, when it got to be stifling. I could get our toothpaste on Tuesday, conveniently forget I needed more Q-tips until Wednesday, save the big trip for seltzer water until Thursday …

Alas. Back in the vet clinic. Numerous owners called around to see if other nearby clinics would subject them to such a terrifying prospect as curbside protocols. It was difficult not to be frustrated. Did they not understand the gravity of what was happening in the world? At least in my small town, all the veterinary facilities were pretty much on the same page, roughly at the same time. I don't know if any clients traveled further in search of someplace else that would coddle their anxiety. For the record, of the nervous clients that did show up with some last-minute begging because Sniffles wouldn't do well without them at their side, guess what? The vast majority of the time, Sniffles and company did *better* without their helicopter owner. Nervous behavior in humans makes animals nervous. Confident handling is far more reassuring. That's not rocket science.

One of my clients wasn't so concerned about the handling of her cats. She trusted us fine for that. But she couldn't bear that she was no longer allowed to come inside for the social half-hour with her favorite veterinarian.

The older woman who had been a consistently good client for years quickly reverted to a childish tantrum in our doorway. I'd planted myself at the entrance, prepared for the hand-off of her cat carrier. When I didn't graciously step aside, she called out to anyone in the lobby that might hear.

"Oh, please, please let us come in! Pull-eeease?"

I admit to being horrified at the display. The cringeworthy begging went on for a bit. Adding that she needed to use our restroom, so we might as well give in anyway. The veterinarian did try to kindly explain to her what the COVID protocol was about. Attempting to smooth things over, but she was still miffed at her frosty reception by the rest of us.

"Well, I'll just have to tell Uncle Billy how I've been treated here today," she declared. Still in an oddly chipper voice. It was the only tone I ever heard from her. A high pitched, typically happy voice. It was almost as if she didn't know how to adjust it to properly express her umbrage. I don't honestly recall which relative of hers she threatened to tell on us, but we'll stick with Uncle Billy. Never met him. Nor could I say why we ought to have felt threatened by him, other than also potentially earning his poor opinion.

Whoever her Uncle Billy was, bless him. I ought to shake the man's hand.

She really did complain, and while I have no idea what was said, he put her in her place. Must have shamed her for acting like a spoiled brat. She'd changed her tune the next time we saw her, and she even conceded that Billy had convinced her this virus was a bigger deal than she wanted to think. From then on, she complied with the curbside rules, for as long as they were in effect. Faithfully dropping off the cats while she ran other errands. Making other restroom arrangements.

Not everyone came around. There would always be those that thought it was ridiculous. Others tried to push past us in the doorway. Whether they didn't think it was a big deal or still thought the virus a hoax. Like our old pal, Preacher. The religious leader in his community, who eventually spat his disgust at us for offending his political sensibilities. His tenure as a client with us ended there. Others pushed for laxity in our standards. Friends or family of staff abused the rules to come in for impractical reasons. Some clients refused to do curbside and wouldn't make an appointment. Others simply decided to take the year off for annual pet exams, and we had no standing to be upset over it. It was the year of 'better safe than sorry.'

One trend we picked up on was an increased frequency of more subtle concerns. Now, understand, we see concerns every day. *My dog is limping, my cat's eye is swollen shut, I think my guinea pig has an ear infection*, et cetera. That's the norm. But when people were home with their pets all day, every day, they developed a keener sense of when things were off. If you were to write that into the medical record, you might say the patient presented for "ADR." That means 'ain't doing right.' Yes, I'm serious. For when symptoms are vague. Difficult to describe, but the owner knows something is not quite right with their pet. *Franklin's breathing weird. My feral cat itched himself seventeen times yesterday. My Shiba Inu didn't feel like eating her morning cheese.* For better or for worse, owners' observation skills were much more attuned. Sometimes it was nothing, other times they were better at early detection of what could have become a bigger problem down the road.

—

The community landscape was different, due to what was being called a full pandemic. There was an eerie sense of being in a zombie apocalypse. Minus the zombies. Playgrounds were devoid of children, closed off with yellow tape. Bars and restaurants abandoned. Signage around town by the city council reminded us to stay home as much as possible and wash our hands. The vintage theatre marquee advertised its closed status along with a plea to "BE SAFE, BE HOPEFUL."

That daily struggle was demoralizing for a while. Constantly weighing what was worth the risk. *How important of an exam is it, really?* We were fearful the same way most others were. Everyone was on edge. Worrying about every interaction. Whether we stood too close. Breathed too close. We were a small staff. If one of us got sick, we presumed all of us would follow, and we'd be forced to shut down.

We watched it happen around town, and in the news. Anxiously awaiting updates of each recorded symptom from the cases trickling into public awareness. Gossip simmering over who in the community had become sick with COVID-19, and what shameful behavior they must have engaged in to catch it. Where did they get it? Did they go out of town? Did they have a social gathering? Suspicions abounded. How old were they and did they have the pre-existing conditions that made them more susceptible? How quickly would the next person get it? What family members should we fear for?

By now it's expected most everyone has caught COVID-19 or one of its variants. At least once, if not more. But at the beginning, it felt as though we looked down on the first to fall sick. Like a scarlet letter wouldn't have been out of order. Folks were ashamed to admit they caught it. Stigmatized.

Coping with stress and exhaustion became crucial. I wasn't unique in that. And joined the rest of America as we sought entertainment and distraction from the depressing news cycle. Political opinions and discourse over the severity of the virus still caused tension, but the country was united through our Netflix accounts. The *Tiger King* documentary about rival wildlife sanctuaries captured everyone for its outrageous twists and turns. The fucked-up antiheroes we all needed in a dark time. The rollercoaster of reality seemed a little less severe when you found out Joe Exotic and his nemeses existed.

Husband and I used to watch the drama unfold while working on our new puzzle hobby every night. We'd think less about coronavirus if we could keep our hands and mind occupied with a few thousand puzzle pieces.

My husband said later it was the first time in our marriage he really worried about my mental state, about how depressed and despairing I often felt. I wanted to help in some way, but didn't know how. Other than going to work, but that didn't feel like it was making any kind of difference. Your daily routine doesn't feel heroic.

When I didn't have a distraction in front of me, I kept thinking more about PPE shortages. Researching major hotspots affected by coronavirus, I started wondering. What did they need?

Following the rabbit hole, I found seamstresses, scientists, and celebrities all working together to endorse homemade masks. Healthcare workers were begging for masks in desperation. Among online groups, there was sharing of patterns and best-case-scenario supplies to use. Dish towels, cotton-blend shirts, vacuum bags, pillowcases, and silk were all household items up for consideration. There was a clear winner ahead of those, if you could find it. Non-woven polypropylene became part of my regular vocabulary, as I began seeking the desired material. Most accessibly, it was a common liner for reusable shopping bags.

I found the two bags I owned. Shoved in a closet for the rare instances I remembered to grab them for shopping. I deconstructed the bags. Requested a free sewing pattern from an online forum and took that guide to work to discuss with an assistant who had sewing skill.

Let it be said, we approached homemade masks fully understanding they could not live up to medical-grade standards. We used the best materials we had. Healthcare workers knew that. Some protection was better than none, though. When the inundated medical world was in a dire enough situation to beg for home-sewn masks, what was the harm in trying? For a time, even the CDC sanctioned their use.

The assistant made two masks. They weren't comfortable, but they looked good and accomplished much of our goal. Fitting needed some kinks worked out, but I credit her for a marvelous first attempt. I started seeking someone to help create more. I didn't have a sewing machine but hoped if I did all the material prep work, that I could find someone willing to sew the final product. A silly ask, in retrospect.

While my inquiry for a willing seamstress resulted in crickets, I got a nudge from a friend. "Just borrow my sewing machine," she said. She'd received one for Christmas years prior and had never taken it out of the box.

My mother used to keep a sewing machine. It was almost always out of commission, though. Tangled threads bunched around the knobs. Abandoned. As a kid, I thought it was fun to play with. Prettily colored threads and a foot pedal to step on. I'd never actually used it.

Needles to say—get it? Needles? Needless? Like, a sewing need—never mind. I was intimidated by the machine dropped off on my doorstep. But I'd been publicly asking for materials and had already received some. Stranded at home, friends and neighbors were willing to find their reusable shopping bags and give me extras. Porch drop-offs, the new communication. I needed to follow through. Put up or shut up about it. Reading through dry instructions, I navigated my way around that machine. Eventually, after pep-talks to myself that the first one was for practice and going to be abysmal, I produced the first attempt.

It *was* abysmal. Crooked lines. Pleating pattern poorly sized. Clumps of thread placed over the strings for fear of them getting yanked out.

Still, it was done. My first face mask.

Then came a second. A third. Inconsistent in the trial runs, as well as a mix-and-match of supplies. Got pretty good at taking the machine apart, when threads broke. You learn faster from mistakes. They weren't perfect, but after completing twelve or fifteen, I couldn't help being mildly proud. The initial batch was put into a shoebox on my front doorstep, with a social media post advertising to my small community.

Honor system, I begged. I wasn't going to police the box, but they were available for those at risk due to health.

At the time, that was the only group for whom it was suggested to wear masks. Elderly and immune-compromised. When CDC recommendations expanded to include everyone, I kept going. For everyone I felt responsible for. When my nearest and dearest were taken care of, I consulted with the online forums of sewing crusaders. Lo and behold, organization was happening. First, just word of mouth. Family of healthcare workers, asking on their behalf. *Send masks to this hospital*, they begged, with the address and point of contact.

Then came official registries, seeking help. Structured by state, or facility type. Some had specifications of masks they would accept. Others were desperate for whatever they could get. I wasn't an experienced enough seamstress to do anything special. I'd figured out my one pattern and was only confident enough to stick with it. But I did it consistently, when I wasn't at work. Obsessively. Husband started giving me time limits at the machine, so I'd take a break. My living room was taken over by card tables, patterns, shopping bags in various stages of deconstruction, and piles of masks. They were boiled when finished, hung to dry, and then enclosed as aseptically as possible into bags.

I was slow enough of a sewer that I only made twenty-five to thirty in a batch. Experienced sewers could have knocked that out in a fraction of the time it took me, but at least I was *doing* something. A call to arms.

By mid-April, batches were mailed to needy destinations that most tugged on my heartstrings. Medical offices, veteran or nursing homes, and a Native American reservation. While most days I felt an urgency to keep going, there were times it seemed ridiculous. Hopeless. Working so hard when I didn't have to. Creating masks to ship them off someplace I would never see. Places I would never receive word from. Did my package arrive? Did they help someone vulnerable? All I could do was hope it wasn't wasted effort.

One side project was for a cousin's hospital, where she was a nurse. She asked me for the headband trend that allowed healthcare workers to avoid excess stress on their ears from wearing masks so frequently. Buttons sewn into a soft headband provided a way to loop the elastic ear bands around something else, securing them in place. To give sore ears a break.

I did the mask projects until the end of June. By then, I had exhausted myself and the world was catching up with demands. The need for homemade masks was slowing down. I made somewhere over two hundred in total. Enough for someone who hadn't properly touched a sewing machine before. People came together to make it happen when it was crucially needed. Community porch drop-offs. My older brother sent funds for supplies. My little sister helped coordinate. One friend was a local business owner that gave piles of shopping bags. However, I discovered there was a plastic covering over the material I wanted. The only usable part was the handles. I let her know, offering to return them. She didn't want them back. Not if some small piece could be used. Another mother lode came from my older sister, who received polypropylene bags as promo swag from her husband's company. I reached a point where I asked people to *stop* donating. Inundated and humbly grateful.

—

Meanwhile, in my day-job, services returned little by little. By mid to late 2020, we slowly resumed grooming appointments, but with reduced numbers per day. Drop-off times were made stricter and staggered every fifteen minutes, so all the owners didn't show up at once. We told clients ad nauseum, we wouldn't be judging any of them for the state of their pets' home-haircut attempts for all the months they'd been put off. There were some doozies, definitely, but we pursed our lips and didn't laugh. Bless animal groomers.

Elective surgeries were allowed to comfortably commence around that same time. When the world had enough available supplies for the human world. If we could get the supplies, we were good to go. For a few months, we had a backlog of owners to work through that had been waiting for spays, neuters, dentals, and benign mass removals.

Like the rest of the world, we closely followed the race for a COVID vaccine. Watched the pharmaceutical companies inching closer and closer. I would have bet money it was impossible to have produced a vaccine that was tested and market-ready before the end of 2020. I was glad to be wrong.

Not that we were first in line. I won't forget everyone clamoring to know their place in the queue. Where they stood in the order of priority to receive the first vaccine. An odd thing, to be categorized in such a way. The human medical field and first responders understandably came first. Veterinary workers were somewhere after that. We checked our local announcements every day. Sometimes refreshing it multiple times a day, waiting impatiently for when it would be our turn. The day when we could check the box stating we were eligible to receive it, and then to compete for available appointment slots. My office manager was concerned that if all of us went to get our first vaccine in one go, we might collectively feel too sick to show up to work the next day. I told her, frankly, I didn't care if we had to close the clinic for a day. We'd been through a hellish year. If it was my turn, I was jumping on the opportunity, clinic hours be damned. The public could do without us for a day. I was getting poked with that needle, and I wished the same for all of them.

We didn't all get in on the same day, and it wasn't so drastic we had to close. But never was I more cheerful to be jabbed. It was a surreal, emotional experience to walk into that community building in the line of people, irrationally fearful I would be called out as some sort of clerical mistake and told to leave. Of course that didn't happen. I received my first Moderna vaccine on January 22, 2021. A Midwest snow and ice storm delayed my group's booster appointment, but we got it completed the following month, on February 25th. Whatever symptoms came of the vaccine—in my case, a day of fatigue, sore arm, and a low-grade fever were worth it. After a year of masking up and sanitizers and social distancing and staying home, hearing of death tolls and heartbreaking lingering effects of the illness, the vaccine made us feel absurdly powerful. Invincible, almost. Giddily flirtatious with danger.

Not that things changed immediately. Far from it. A community doesn't spend that long on high alert and then just flip a switch overnight.

We had to still insist on curbside for a while. Calling for consideration and common decency when people pressured for a state of normalcy in public again. We had to remind our clients of that, too, when they complained.

"I can't come in? This is bullshit. I've been vaccinated!"

"Yes, but *I* haven't yet!" the manager had to say more than once.

The process of vaccinating everyone happened in stages. I was relatively lucky to get in so early. Husband didn't get his until March. Other friends and acquaintances were in the last community group, of lowest medical or working risk. They didn't get their chance until summer. One thing I never got tired of, in that time was celebrating anyone when it was their turn. When they texted or posted their social media selfies with glee. I made my father's appointment for him, as he was my biggest concern for being medically-compromised if he were to catch COVID. The moment I found out he was in an eligible group, I filled out the confusing registration forms for him, then called him and told him where to go. I was thrilled the day our family group message thread received his blurry, badly-composed photo of him with a sticker that announced he'd been vaccinated, near the end of March.

Coming back out of curbside service was something we did gradually. Our main part-time assistant had moved on to another job during 2020, and the two new young hires that replaced her had never even worked in our facility when clients were allowed to be *inside* the building. We were out of practice, and I'm sure they were completely intimidated to have to talk to someone from behind the lobby counter the first time.

I'll admit there was a freedom to not letting the public into our clinic. Exams in 2020 were more efficient because we could do the job without having to slow down to explain to the client what was happening. Explanations and discussion were saved for the parking lot. Inside, we could speak more freely, certainly, without the owner standing right there. It might not be shocking to know myself and few other staff members, including the vets, had gotten too comfortable with letting profanity loose. Professional speech had to be practiced again.

Proclamations such as, "Holy shit, Roscoe got fat!" would have to shift back to, "Mr. Williams, Roscoe is looking a little heavier than we'd like to see. His ideal body weight should be closer to forty-five pounds, and he's currently seventy-two …"

We bought sneeze guards to put up on the counter to ease into the transition. Often still wore masks, for as long as the city council was still recommending them. Signage was posted for when they were required, but it was awkward and difficult to enforce at times. Especially when after some of the staff had been vaccinated, and they too felt they shouldn't have to continue masking up. Harder to enforce rules when your own lead staff isn't setting the example. Eventually, we had to let people do as they chose. A lot of peer pressure went into it, too. Staff and clients alike would many a time be checking out the other to see if masks were worn. An etiquette stand-off, almost. Trying to be considerate and follow the program. While I still saw the rare mask worn months and years after, the protocols were phased out. We took down our sneeze guard one day with the intent to clean it and then replace it. Instead, we just never put it back up. Even that made us feel oddly exposed. The disappearance of a clear piece of plastic seemed to open up the room, and at the same time, bring us into intimate contact with the people standing three feet away. The very next day, a regular client walked in and made negative comments about the guard being gone. She missed the safety of the shield.

Like many others surely experienced, our social anxieties had morphed because of the pandemic. It would be many more months before I felt comfortable standing in a group of people again. I still get stressed out when someone hovers too close in the grocery check-out line. Biting my tongue not to snap at the offender to give me space. The first times Husband

and I ventured out without masks, we felt overly exposed. Nearly scandalous. After a year of spending so much time on our own, I struggle more with friendly social interactions. I was never good at it in the first place, but it's a different kind of challenge, now.

I presume 2020 was not anyone's year. Certainly not mine. The effects of it linger still, years after. They should. For better or for worse, the world ought to have responded to that crisis and made changes. Adapted. It seems foolish to suggest anyone could go back to 2019 and earlier. Spending a year having to prioritize what was essential and what was worth risking safety created a new normal. Navigating how society operated. Trimming the fat of superfluous bullshit. I don't mean to imply that we should do without culture. Without arts or nice things. Those are imperative, and in fact, those were keeping people bonded, united, and hopeful during the darker days. Music, films, theatre, art, writing, and all the homemade crafts. Whether or not talent was apparent in them didn't matter. Those are things worth living for. Adding wonder to our existence.

Nature walks with our beloved pets became more frequent. How many more people got out of their house with their dog and saw beauty on the block where they live? Beauty that might normally have gone ignored, because of all the other fluff we fill our lives with to stay busy? Our pets were heroes that year, keeping people sane at home. Adoptions, rescues, and fosters increased in that time. Friendships may have been better maintained because we had the technology to check in with each other more conveniently. My two best friends lived elsewhere. We had semi-regular video-calls, adult beverages in hand, where we genuinely asked how each other were doing. We didn't do that before. Not on the same scale.

In many ways, the pandemic made community harder to sustain. Being apart from each other and relying on connection through a screen isn't a good long-term solution. Humans need real contact, and the return to connection was not without struggle or strife. There were devastating losses of life because of COVID-19, and terrible hardships on businesses, finances, economy, sufferers from other chronic illnesses outside of the virus whose care was put on the backburner, and both emotional and physical strain on people's lives.

It's not up to me to determine what everyone ought to take from that difficult time, but for me, it honed my priorities. Unnecessary drama is discouraged from my life. I try to do better telling family and friends I appreciate them. Slowly but surely, I'm chipping away at that list of things I always wanted to do.

Superstitious

"Superstition is the religion of feeble minds."
—Edmund Burke

I'm not a superstitious human by nature. Alas, there are superstitious rules one abides by when they've done this veterinary business long enough. The fact that we have years of scientific training and background is irrelevant. Respect the rules.

I present them in no particular order. Nor do they really require further explanation.

- Naming your pet "Lucky" is the unluckiest name you can give them. Tragedy befalls the poor bastards. Don't do it.
- If the collar says "Sweetie," "Precious," or some other sugar-inspired name, be careful with your digits! Don't get bitten. In contrast, if it's a "Killer," "Cujo," or "Brutus," you're probably in for some adorable cuddles.
- Don't ever say, "Kind of a slow day, huh?" In some clinics, "quiet" is a dirty word.
- Don't buy your old pet a new collar. Bad juju. Only purchase a new one if the old one is irreparably broken. We cringe when we see the shiny new adornment around the neck of your sweet senior dog, certain you've just doomed him to an imminent illness.

- Never comment on how great a vein looks, prior to the attempted venipuncture. Even if it's a hose. Say nothing. I'm known for being respectable at the task, but even I once failed to hit a cow's jugular when the impressive size was remarked upon. A fucking cow, folks ... In my early learning days, I had a running joke with a fellow VA whenever our shifts were aligned. Despite getting along great as humans, we were convinced we were a hex on each other's phlebotomy skills, no matter how great the patient. We deemed ourselves (ironically) "DBDD," for Dynamic Blood-Draw Duo.
- Euthanasia happens in threes. If you hit number four in a week, the cycle starts over again. Two more to go before the week's out. I've once seen us hit nine, which is impressive for a small-town clinic.
- Obscure case conditions also happen in threes. Two years since you've done an aural hematoma repair? Why not do three all at once?
- Get out more equipment than necessary, to ensure you'll be successful on the first attempt. Catheters, needles, trach tubes, whatever. Acting cocky guarantees failure.
- The error-beeping pulse oximeter/blood pressure monitor/fluid pump etc. will start working again once you walk away from it.
- Pouring the exact number of pills needed from the bottle indicates good fortune. Not a bad time to buy a lotto ticket.

Spill the Ampu-Tea

"The purity of a person's heart can be quickly
measured by how they regard animals."
—Theophile Gautier

When I was beating myself up about a case, an older, wiser colleague reminded me of the corny play on words. It's called veterinary *practice* for a reason. Not veterinary perfection.

Sounds dumb as hell, I agree. Doesn't make it less true, though. We'll always be honing the craft. Learning from experiences, literature, and research to do better for the next case. Show me the human who did everything correctly the first time. No? Great.

Because veterinary medicine is not perfect, some methodological practices have fallen out of favor, too. Tail docking, ear cropping, and declawing are some of the procedures under fire. Once widely accepted, they've since come under scrutiny, and for good reason. The former two are frowned upon, if done purely for cosmetic reasons. No longer sanctioned by the AVMA. Banned in some countries, amidst evolving ideas about breed standards.

Are there medical reasons to perform these procedures? Sure. One of the best reasons to dock the coccygeal vertebrae is the condition affectionately known as "happy tail." This occurs when a dog has too much enthusiasm for life, and that overjoyed tail wags so damn hard that it hits walls or hard surfaces, causing injuries upon injuries to the poor anatomical indicator of bliss. Honestly, is there anything better than such a condition in a species? What other ailment has joy in the description? Never mind the constant open wounds flinging blood spatter everywhere. The wagging doesn't stop in those doggos. Thus, in the case of happy tail syndrome, amputating the greater length of the tail is often seen as a saving measure against recurrent injury. Most common in short-haired, larger breeds with muscular tails.

Ear cropping, like tail docking, was primarily for breed aesthetics and standardizing. It was once thought there was additional medical benefit of preventing ear infections, but that argument doesn't hold up so well anymore, either. Thankfully I didn't have to help with many of these procedures, but heard it requested. Mostly from older folks, wanting it for their Schnauzers to appear sharp and distinguished. Or, from the other end of the spectrum, many wanted their muscle dogs to appear menacing. And it felt gross to do.

You may recall from the dreaded Breeds chapter, our ear cropping clients. Well, they sucked. As I saw it, they were seeking an illusion of power, via their canines. A tough status symbol. For themselves, or to sell to like-minded individuals. They didn't give a shit about vaccines or any other preventive veterinary medicine. No money for that nonsense. All they wanted was an aesthetic. We got tired of performing the surgery for those people.

With the practice becoming less respectable and rarer to find via safe methods, I hate to report that we heard of nightmare home surgeries. Guys that would perform a botched procedure on their dogs in their kitchens at home. Suturing up the mess with a plain old sewing needle and thread. Our vet saw one such dog after the wounds got infected. Go figure. Another client was dismayed when our receptionist told him over the phone that we no longer conducted ear crops. He admitted to her that because he couldn't find a vet to do it anymore, he was gearing up to do it himself. She sternly reminded him such an undertaking wasn't legal. He hung up quickly after that.

As an aside, while we elected to stop doing the procedure, it was one that required some finesse and technique to do it well and correctly. Ain't just a straightforward hack job. Ears badly cut, whether by legal means or not, set the dogs up for health problems later.

There will always be rare medical exceptions to endorse such procedures. Usually, though, we err in favor of keeping these mentioned regions of anatomy.

Now, for the toes.

When I say declawing, I'm going to be referring to the procedure for cats. Yes, dogs will sometimes go through removal of a *dew*claw (note the spelling difference), but that practice usually has practical purpose. Especially in more active breeds who risk tearing a dewclaw during activity. But I digress—we're not talking dewclaws. We're talking *de*claws. In cats.

The fancy name for the procedure is an onychectomy. It's what folks put their feline friends through for the sake of peaceful cohabitation in their domiciles. Usually, an attempt to save their bourgie furniture from getting clawed up. Some debate used to exist around the preferred methods of doing the cutting during the procedure (scalpel vs trimmers vs lasers), but the result was the same: the removal of the distal phalanges (the last bone) in each toe, along with the attached nail. Sometimes, just a portion of that bone was removed.

Complications from declawing can certainly happen. Acute or chronic pain in the feet. Lameness. Infections. Worsened arthritis later in life. Plenty of others.

One of the big-ticket items is the behavioral standpoint. Scratching is a natural behavior for a cat, whether for a good stretch or to express excitement or anxiety. Removing the claws eliminates their ability to do it effectively. Even in a litterbox, scratching around to pick a location or to cover up their mess may be more painful.

Aggression often creeps in for a declawed cat. Tons of my clients thought they'd be doing a good thing by removing claws to avoid being scratched. Instead, they sometimes created a worse problem. Why? One of kitty's main lines of defense had been taken away, causing them to be more vulnerable. No claws to throw out a good warning swat. What's left to them, when they feel threatened or upset? Increased aggression, and teeth. I always worried more when a family wanted a good lap-cat for their aging Nana and thought they'd do her thin skin a favor by declawing the animal. The intentions were thoughtful, but not thought-out.

I don't want to cause shame to folks that weren't aware of the severity of problems a declaw can cause, nor to those who have kitties that have undergone the procedure. Hell, our own clinic cats were front-declawed. Many of our cat-loving staff quietly admitted they'd have had a difficult time being cat owners were it not for declawing. Hypocritical feelings aside, as the world started reassessing this practice, we were all in agreement. If an owner couldn't deal with this natural aspect of the animal, perhaps cat ownership was not the best thing for them.

It wasn't a decision that happened overnight. The onychectomy procedure is still legal in most states, but the pressure was there. The AVMA eventually came out against it. While that doesn't mean it's banned and clinics have to stop, it was certainly becoming frowned upon. Some states and other countries had banned it already, and I expected the trend to continue.

With the topic up for discussion in my clinic, I printed out guides and explanations of the dying practice for my VAs to have for reference, so they could understand the debate and what our responsibility was. As a clinic, we agreed that with the controversial practice going the direction that it was, we were going to get stricter on our existing protocols. We only allowed for a short window of time during the developing kitten period to do the procedure. A few weeks at just the right time, to prevent further complications. Exceptions had been made in the past, but no more. When folks called asking about it for their three-year-old cat, we had to remember not to rudely laugh at them. Sorry, long overdue and too late.

An older or bigger cat would have far worse barriers to recovery. Off-limits.

As the number of these procedures decreased in our clinic's schedule, I realized I wasn't missing it, whatsoever. It was a stressful process and hard on the patients, for what had always seemed, in the back of my mind, a selfish reason to do it. Let's be honest, I never gave a fuck what clients spent on their designer couch. If they threw a cheap blanket over the armrest, maybe that would spare the feline from mutilated paws. And here, our governing body was handing us the golden-ticket excuse to stop.

The vets were of the same mind. Our strict standards became not just that, but also a tentative deadline. After a certain date, we dared to suggest we were going to be done with declawing altogether. There were just a few lingering appointments on the books that had been promised.

It was me that fucked up.

Before that end date was reached, I took the call from one of our regular clients, who had a new kitten. I was soon reminded that both their older cats had had all four feet declawed. Which is a bit unusual. Most vets stick to the front feet only. But this cat-loving couple was eager to incorporate their newest into the family tradition.

I tried to express my hesitation. Maybe even a little bit of guilt-tripping to get her to reconsider. Understandably, she had questions. I explained patiently why we were phasing out declawing and becoming extremely strict on who we still performed the surgery for. The countdown of removing the service from our list. Idiot that I was, I pretty much blabbed the magic words to say, in justifying our limitations of the age-appropriate kitten window AND for clients who had medical concerns about getting scratched-up. You know. Folks on blood-thinners and whatnot.

As soon as it was out of my mouth, I knew I shouldn't have said it.

She hung up from that phone call, stating she needed to speak with her husband. And wouldn't you know it? A few hours later when she called back, husband had a medical condition that required him to be on blood-thinners! The odds, right?

Kitten was scheduled not just for two paws, but to add insult, they requested all four feet to be declawed. The appointment came, and it was done. I was seething with resentment about their duplicitousness, but I couldn't easily accuse them of being full of shit.

In the recovery ward later that morning, I stood with my arms crossed over my chest. An unpleasant churning in my stomach, observing my poor little patient. Mewling. Stumbling. Pathetically trying to hold herself upright. Sure, she was still a bit groggy from anesthesia. But that didn't change the fact that she had four legs of thick bandages she could hardly stand in. Frustrated. Undeservedly struggling to get over the lip of the litter box, or to reach her water bowl without clumsily tipping it over.

The vet came and stood next to me, observing the same. Both of us were quiet for a few moments, listening to the kitten's distress. She would heal up in time, but it was cold comfort to this traumatic moment.

"I don't want to do it anymore," I said.

"No," he agreed. "I don't think I do, either."

That was the last onychectomy our clinic performed. The closing window snapped shut.

Looking for Answers

"Questions are never indiscreet, answers sometimes are."
—Oscar Wilde

There is comfort in a diagnosis.

An answer. An explanation. Humans are curious creatures. If we don't know the logic of the what, where, or why, we're inclined to make up a hypothesis. Or a story. Something to explain the looming question. What is it? Where did it originate? Why did it happen?

A handful of times in my career, the veterinary team has hit a wall. The patient's illness, a mystery. Symptoms, elusive. Lab results, inconclusive. And that bothers us. Makes us feel like failures, for the ones that don't seem to quite fit into a category. They don't follow the textbook guidelines to explain what's wrong.

Sometimes even if we do figure out what's wrong, it doesn't change the outcome of what happens with the pet. The attempted therapy may have been the same. Or maybe the pet is still headed toward the same inevitable end. Yet the owners appreciate understanding *why* it's happening. To make an informed decision, because they could at least put a name to the culprit.

Sometimes we've simply run out of time. The patient was too far gone, and we had to let them go before we could solve the puzzle. It happens. Plenty of other times, we had to be content with our list of possible rule-outs, due to working within the parameters of the owner's finances. They couldn't afford the diagnostic tests to determine if it was X-organ failure, Y-cancerous process, or Z-immune disorder. These scenarios happen on a semi-frequent basis.

But those rare ones do exist. Where we have the funds to seek the answers. Where we ought to have had sufficient time. And yet, an answer isn't found.

One of the supervisors of a practice where I worked had such a dog. I was still brand new to the field during this case. Outdoor, middle-aged, male sporting breed dog started to drop weight and experience periods of lethargy and inappetence. To be honest, I can't remember all the symptoms now. I couldn't tell you what was on the rule-out list. Dysautonomia, probably, for its unclear symptoms. Maybe a tick-borne pathogen, or an immune disorder. Some other rare virus. What I do know is that for numerous weeks, the supervisor had to keep bringing the dog back to her own place of work. More diagnostics. More trial therapies for the abstract illness. She gave him time. She gave him resources. She dropped several hundred dollars or more to try to determine what was causing her beloved dog to become weaker and thinner and unrecognizable.

After a time, enough was enough, and she couldn't bring herself to put him through any more. She and her husband made the heartbreaking call to end his suffering. What I will never forget is going to let the attending veterinarian know that she and her family awaited him in the exam room, at their appointed time. This time, as the client, rather than as our fellow staff member. They had said their goodbyes and were ready for the vet to come in with the necessary drugs.

"*I'm* not ready," the vet answered me. And I realized, he needed another minute to compose himself. To dash away the tears brimming in his eyes so he could be the brave one in the room.

I will never forget the other vets sending her messages of condolence when it was done.

"I'm so sorry that we couldn't even give you a diagnosis," said one.

Sometimes our knowledge and our tests have limitations. We can't fix everything. It feels like failure. Like we should have been able to figure it out. Or do something more. Sometimes we must accept we did all we could do in a situation.

Ambiguity is a romantic notion for the creatives in us. Great for art and writing and theatrical pursuits. Shades of gray that dabble in possibilities. What does the painting represent to you? What did the film ending mean? On the flipside, ambiguity does not sit well for the scientific brains. Black and white answers, please, for the logic-craving crowd. It is, or it isn't. Yes or no.

Sometimes we're determined that we know the answer, even if the evidence isn't supporting it. Doggedly obstinate about the theory. If mange is suspected in a patient, the dermatological test we reach for first is a simple skin scrape. Easily done in practice. With a dulled scalpel blade, one literally scrapes the skin of the patient where lesions are present, wipes that residue on a prepared slide, and then searches for evidence of the pesky mites under the microscope. It doesn't hurt the patient as badly as it sounds. There's some technique to it.

In any case, it's a good starting test, but it's not the most reliable test. Patients can be positive for mange, but sometimes you can't find the mites for proof. One of my supervising doctors would groan after I announced "negative" as I rolled through the entirety of the slide.

"Scrape them again!"

And so we would, as many times as felt acceptable. Seeking that definitive answer.

Or the constant dietary indiscretion cases. We see numerous diarrhea-episode patients with an indecisive history. Owner doesn't know what's different. No apparent stressors, no food changes, no new treats, no toddlers dumping food on the kitchen floor to explain what the dog might have gotten into. No evidence of raiding trash or eating miscellaneous things from the yard. We're just left with an annoying symptom in a dog that seems otherwise fine. Still bright and alert. Not vomiting, usually.

After running all the fecal tests, if it's negative for parasites, and all we see is the expected bacterial overgrowth on a cytology, the doctor will usually diagnose the disappointingly vague "colitis" or "gastrointestinal enteritis." Then send home the generic antibiotics with accompanying probiotics. Depending on the doctor's philosophy, maybe a few days' worth of prescription bland food.

If symptoms persisted and the diarrhea came back, the frustrated owners returned. We considered more in-depth diagnostics. Bloodwork or GI scopes, or ... and then we remembered. Wait, have we ruled out giardia yet?

Extremely difficult to detect in a standard fecal exam, this little bastard of a prion parasite gets an exam of its own. We convince the owner to let us run that annoyingly specific test for that one parameter. Nine times out of ten, it's negative, too. So, we carry on with our other diagnostics. But guys, when the elusive line shows up as a positive for giardia? It's the Super Bowl (in our case, the Puppy Bowl) for the veterinary staff. The doctor is high fiving me and we're doing hushed whoops and a quiet victory dance, so the owner doesn't hear us in the lab and wonder what kind of demented buffoon celebrates a parasite.

Why? Because it's so specific, and the treatment, so definite. We know. We know exactly what it is. A giardia parasite! Giardiasis! Beaver fever (yep, for real)! We can consult the book on the recommended medication regimen. It's a clear-cut, convenient answer for the no-longer frustrating puzzle. Tie it up and put a bow on it.

There is comfort in that diagnosis.

For the Sake of Levity: Overreaction

It was very late, and the exhausted team looked forward to closing time. For me, probably to eat an obscene number of nachos, drink a piss-water beer, do the bare minimum of studying for tomorrow's Clin-Path quiz, and call it a night while falling asleep to sitcom re-runs. Others may have had something more dignified, but I was the lonely college kid then.

The last thing we wanted was a hysterical phone call from a good client just before the end of the day. That's what we got. Owner had discovered a mass on her beloved cat while petting her and was absolutely beside herself with fear. The dreaded C-word?

Receptionist told her to come on in and we'd take a look, before calling it a night. She showed up in a mess of tears, devastated at the thought of what would become of her sweet kitty.

To this day, I still wonder whether our receptionist charged an additional emergency fee for our veterinarian to tell her the diagnosis: fat.

The cat was just damned fat. No tumor, no mass, not even a lipoma, which is a benign fatty mass … just … plain fat.

Owner probably learned what a primordial pouch was that evening. I'm sure it was an expensive education.

What's It Take?

"Success is not final; failure is not fatal: it is the courage to continue that counts."
—Winston Churchill

I'm not the authority on qualities that make one a success in the field. All I can give is my humble perception of helpful traits as a veterinary professional. Nothing you wouldn't expect.

Curiosity to keep you engaged with your cases. Research is essential to a developing science, one in which we learn more all the time. That's what continuing education requirements are for, but apart from fulfilling annual requirements to check off a license form, a professional ought to *want* to learn more about the subjects that intrigue them. Be a proud nerd.

Creativity is a plus. Or you could swap that word for resourcefulness. Because of the uniqueness of cases, you sometimes have to be flexible. Often, medicine is not made for animals. Vets are very familiar with the concept of extra-label use, when there is no existing medication tailor-made for the species being treated, for the specific problem it's having. They'll seek reference literature or other guides to recommend what closest approximation would be safe, and dosage protocols. This is an especially common occurrence for exotic patients. There's just not a lot of money in production of medicine for guinea pigs or rabbits. Little market for it. And why would there be? It's cheaper to replace your hamster than to treat the sick one. Trust me, that's the route most parents of young children choose. Point is, you might have to get creative in your treatment of the lizard that doesn't have a precise rulebook to accompany its care. Or when equipment doesn't fit your animal. Inventing contraptions to serve as an Elizabethan collar (e-collar, for short; or, cone of shame) is a handy skill. Or fashioning a splint out of tongue depressors to fit the leg of the tiny kitten weighing less than two pounds.

I've already ranted about communication. We like our animals, and we like the privilege of being their voice, but we have to communicate with the humans that own them. Bedside manner, being approachable and sympathetic to client concerns all fall under this umbrella. Not only that but keeping harmony with your team. Talk, as needed. That includes good cooperation skills. No one can pull off veterinary work alone, so if someone's trying to be the action hero, too tough and jaded to need help from anyone, that ego's going to crash and burn. Medicine is a better place without egos.

Observational skills were harped about in another section, so we won't beat that dead horse. But that's crucial to good care of your patients and record-keeping.

Some manner of organization is a plus. I'm not the tidiest person in the world, but I have a system and I hate when it's disrupted. My assistants sometimes ask if they can reorganize my surgery room, in a way that I may reluctantly admit makes more sense to the flow of operations. Still, I'm stubbornly slow to accept those changes. If they want to move the cup containing my bandage scissors three feet to the left on the countertop, I command that it be done incrementally. Otherwise, when I reach for those scissors and they're not in the location I expect them to be, I get irritated. Probably something undiagnosed there, but … meh. We'll leave it. Point is, there's value in organized consistency, as long as it's not chaotic to the rest of the team.

Advocating for patients, teammates, and yourself. Another horse we can spare from further violence, so let's be brief. It takes a strong—but level—person to know when to step up. What battles to pick. When to bite your tongue. How you want to be treated, quality of care you provide, and when to draw lines? All things to be evaluated. A strong sense of ethical responsibility goes with this. You may need to learn the rules and regulations to be followed, but one ought to have a sense of principles in place already.

Sense of humor is crucial. I'm no comedian and burdened with the shameful condition of loving a good pun. But if you've been diligently reading through these stories, all the levity moments, and haven't once chuckled or even cracked a smile? Maybe you've figured out thirty pages ago, veterinary life is perhaps not for you. You have to find humor in this job, or you'll hate it. Despair in it. If you can find comic relief from others' descriptions and my telling ain't your cup of tea, all well and good. Just make sure you laugh, if you've plunged into this. Humor is what will help you to persist when things get tough. When it gets too serious.

I once had a client traveling to Canada for a short visit, who wanted to be allowed to take her pet sugar glider. She asked our help to make sure she had the necessary documentation to permit its entry across the border. After an hour of intensive research, including making calls to Canadian offices that didn't appreciate my appalling lack of French-speaking ability, I felt certain I was the world's foremost expert in requirements for an American citizen crossing into Canada with a *Petaurus breviceps*. Don't ask me anymore, as I've long since forgotten. But it's laughably absurd.

As was the time I urgently texted my VA coworker before her afternoon shift: *"Don't come to work yet! I'll clock ya in but need you to run an errand first. Call me."* That errand entailed her driving to the local hospital (the human one) parking lot, weaving through the rows of parked vehicles, until she found the one containing poor Rue and Rowdy. Our regular canine patients waited anxiously in the owner's truck, after the owner had driven himself to hospital. Recognizing he was feeling the effects of a heart attack, he wasn't going to leave his beloved dogs home alone. However, the crotchety old cuss of a man (lotta bark, no bite—can you tell I adored him?) wouldn't submit to any treatment, until his nurse called our clinic first. She did, begging us for help with the unorthodox rescue mission. The thankfully-sweet-tempered dogs were retrieved and safely boarded at our facility. I called the nurse back with the green light. Even more thankfully, the owner later recovered and was able to reclaim his dogs.

If you can't find amusement in your day-to-day, then I don't know what more you want.

Multilingual skills help, as they would in any industry. I can't guarantee I can hold a conversation in any foreign language I've dabbled in, but it is quite fun to be able to explain what a patellar luxation is in Spanish. Or that their pet has intestinal worms. Or even to stumble through grooming instructions.

I've even picked up a tiny amount of sign language for a few symptoms. It's pretty obvious when I need translation help, but making the effort goes a long way for clients for whom English is a second language.

A strong stomach. That should be a no-brainer, but it's worth mentioning again. When first considering the career, I shadowed at a few clinics to see if it was my jam. The staff allowed me to observe a Labrador being spayed, and I felt the panic that probably many people would if they'd never seen live surgery before. *Will I panic? Faint? Vomit?* The procedure started mid-morning and my gag reflex remained unaffected. Much to my surprise, halfway through the fascinating process, my stomach growled.

Ooh, lunch time is coming up, I thought to myself.

I was staring into the open body cavity of a dog and meanwhile wondering which bread bowl I would order from Panera across the parking lot, in the very near future. That told me what I needed to know. Broccoli cheddar was the clear winner … Oh, and squeamishness wouldn't be a problem for me.

Not usually. I often joke that my biggest failing as an RVT is handling ticks. More times than I would prefer, I've felt a patient's skin tag under my fingers. Only to look down and realize I'm not fondling a skin tag, but an engorged tick. That starts the gag reflex. Followed by the swift urge to bleach my hand. I despise those little bastards, and any request to remove ticks from a pet is a request I'll pass along to anybody but me. There. Now you know my worst quality. Ticks make me fall apart. Other than being food for some ground birds, they're the most worthless insect to the ecosystem. Utterly villainous.

So, if I've listed the good qualities, it stands to reason to mention the opposites. Folks on the other end of those spectrums are going to have a harder time of things. You're all smart enough to figure out what those opposite qualities would be, so let's just give you the tough examples I've come across in the wild—er, in the field.

We hired a young man as a VA once, a pre-vet major, no less, who lasted less than three months. Looked good on paper, but I should have paid attention to his subtle negative attitude when he showed up during pandemic curbside service to drop off his resumé and I didn't allow him inside. He'd already started another clinic job, but since our hours of need didn't conflict, we were ok with the concurrent position. However, another alarm bell was set off when he described his other boss to us, mentioning that veterinarian had sworn he would never write him a letter of reference, so he was hoping ours would, when the time came. Didn't sound like a joke. An odd threat to make to someone still under your employment. We never got a chance to speak to the other vet for his side of the story, but something didn't add up.

Eager-to-please is not always a bad thing to start, but this VA had an outward ego I suspect was a cover for deep insecurity. Tried too damn hard to fake perfection, and instead just showed the fake. That doesn't work in medicine. It's an environment that calls for honesty and humility. Ego has no room when it comes to the care of something other than yourself.

Our relief vet and I were rechecking a rectal tumor case one morning. This involved a rectal exam, of course, on a very nice American bully. Vet palpated it first, and as she trusts my opinion, wanted me to take a turn for the area of concern. It would be a very elusive nodule, and subtle difference in texture compared to surrounding tissue, she advised me. Also, it might take a minute to be certain of the right area. Following her directions, I felt for the nodule. She was right. It wasn't immediately obvious. I had to keep running my fingers along the surface several times. After thirty or forty seconds, there it was. I agreed with her assessments.

Having watched this whole process, the vet then offered for our VA to have a turn. Learning opportunity, why not? He gloved up, and I watched as he began.

Within three seconds he said, "Oh, yeah. I feel it."

"... Do you?" the vet asked, and then clarified what he should be feeling.

He affirmed, but then he couldn't hide the moment where it was legit, about thirty seconds later. When he *actually* felt what he was supposed to feel. His eyes dilated.

The "Oooh," moment.

That brief exchange bothered the hell out of me. That someone would be competitive about something so ridiculous as how quickly he detected a mass, lying to improve his optics in the situation. If he would lie about such a petty thing, what bigger issues would come along?

I recalled vividly in tech school, one of my classmates asking for help from the instructor during a lab. The task was differentiating parasite species under the microscope, two of which looked extremely similar to one another. I overheard the instructor explaining what structures she should be seeking through the lens. Student peered into it. Paused. Adjusted her microscope settings and looked again. With dismay, said, "I'm not seeing it."

"What?" the instructor replied. "Really? Let me fix your lighting ..."

She made another adjustment, and the classmate looked once more. Several moments passed.

"I'm sorry, I just don't see it," classmate finally admitted. The instructor was taken aback, but she found herself faced with a student that visually couldn't discern the defining characteristic of the specimen she was meant to see. That was an important component to the lesson, and in retrospect, I appreciate the humility it must have taken to admit to it. She could have lied or cheated on her test. But she wasn't going for a competition. Not for ego. She was learning the information for the good of her future patients.

In our clinic, though, the VA's most egregious moment came about while trying to keep the client happy. A pet was dropped off to be groomed one morning and was meant to have his annual vaccinations, too. Either the staff missed the memo, or just got busy. Bottom line, the dog didn't get the vaccines. When the owner came to pick up the dog, the doctor was already on an extended lunch break. I'm not sure what happened in that exchange between our VA and the client, but in his version, the client was upset and didn't want to make another trip. So, you probably guessed.

VA took it upon himself to fully vaccinate the dog, issue the yearly license, and send them on their way.

It's a heinous no-no, if you're at all unsure. That's something only a licensed vet is authorized to do, and even I, as an RVT, am bound by constraints on how much I can do without the vet being present, or without express permission.

I was livid when I found out, and shocked someone with prior veterinary experience didn't know that. Maybe their rules at the other clinic were too lax? I tried not to lose my cool when I sat him down for the discussion, but I'm sure he could tell I was pissed. It came down to ethical integrity, I reminded him. He hoped to one day earn the DVM role for himself, and in my mind, already had an at-risk reputation. That client's pet didn't get a qualified exam from its doctor that year. I told the VA that I would rather he risk pissing off the client, than risk his status as a trustworthy professional. It reflected poorly on him and even worse on the clinic's character. Client might have been annoyed at the moment, but a reasonable person would have eventually understood. Some discount could have been offered to appease them. If they were still going to be upset after that, they weren't worth hanging onto as a client.

I won't lie when I say I wanted to fire the VA there and then, but was overruled. It was decided he had another chance. Alas, I don't think he even made it through the following weekend. Once before, he'd made an excuse about his alarm clock breaking and hoping the sunlight through the window would wake him up from the living room sofa. We didn't believe that excuse for his tardiness, but it wasn't as if we could prove him wrong.

This time, once again, he failed to show on time for his solo Saturday work shift. No doctor staffed that day for appointments. It was a morning available for clients to pick up scripts and for boarded animals to be taken care of. The manager happened to be stopping by the clinic to pick something up, half an hour after the office was meant to be open. When she arrived, the parking lot was empty, lights in the building off, and the door locked. Now it was her turn to be livid. It hadn't been her plan to work that shift, but nonetheless, found herself covering it. Taking boarded dogs outside to relieve bladders first, followed by a late breakfast.

VA came screeching into the lot about ten minutes later, hoping no one would notice he was then forty minutes late for his shift.

She furiously demanded his key and told him he was fired. Soon I found out I wasn't the only one relieved at his forced departure, but for one notable exception.

The few men that are present in veterinary medicine always revel in the excitement when they have another male coworker, as they're normally constantly surrounded by women. The veterinarian brought it up a few times during the following weeks, whether we ought to give the kid one more chance? He missed the camaraderie. Someone that could hold a conversation about football, hunting, or whatever. The manager and I shut him down sharply. We didn't want to work with that VA anymore. Too many occasions demonstrating lack of integrity.

He wouldn't earn a reference letter from any of our staff, either, it turned out. Maybe he'll mature and be more ready for the medical field in years to come. I don't know, but until he does, someone with such questionable judgment is not fit.

We once hired a girl who was perfectly nice, but, I suspect, was pushed into applying by a parent who thought it might be a future career lead for her.

During her interview, she'd asked about dress code. Good question. I'd shown her the scrub tops she had at her disposal from the clinic, to wear during her shift. Otherwise, close-toed shoes and long pants. Scrub pants or jeans fine, so long as they weren't holey jeans, like one would wear at a rock concert. Potential for them to get snagged during restraint of an animal.

She showed up on her first day with shredded jeans. I chose not to say anything about that immediately, but told her to go pick out a scrub top and then find me in the lab. She came out in her own sports-themed t-shirt.

The first thought in my mind was, *Is she defiant, or …?*

I reiterated the instruction about the scrub top.

"Oh, it's fine, I'll just wear this," she said cheerily enough.

I shook my head. "No, I mean ... I need you to wear one of those shirts. Protects you working with patients, protects your own clothes, identifies you as an employee ...? You know?"

"Oh, ok!"

Ok. Pleasant enough. Not defiant. It was the alternative. I worried.

It was soon clear she was in over her head. I like it when new personnel take the initiative to ask questions about the cases they see. On the rare occasion this girl did, there was nothing wrong with the questions, per se, but they were not at the depth of someone who has more interest in the field. In addition, even minor processes were shocking to her. She gasped the first time she saw a patient's temperature taken rectally. If that was alarming, it was going to get a lot worse.

I didn't need her on a surgery shift, but I started encouraging her to observe a couple of routine procedures anyway. Same as it was for me, it might give some indication whether she had the stomach for this. Make or break moment. If she showed interest in any of the processes or anatomy. Even with initial hesitation, if they can take a moment and then persevere, that's telling.

We later employed a VA who's great about most everything. Meticulous, compassionate, and eager. Until suturing. Her knees get shaky at this point of a procedure. The rest is fine, but the needlework makes her squeamish. We can work around that, when everywhere else in the clinic, she's a solid worker and smart as hell.

For our less-invested hire, if the girl's instinct was to run screaming from the surgical suite, that was going to be a problem in the long run. Fact is, I needed someone who wasn't going to fall apart when an emergency walked in the door. A hit-by-car, or a necrotic wound, for example. Or any bodily fluids. At some point, she would need to handle a syringe.

About that time, I was sure missing another previous long-time great VA who had gotten pregnant and left for a different career path. She wasn't, and didn't ever have to be a veterinary student, but she was one of the best. I could fondly recall a canine patient we'd sat on the floor with, together. Ignoring the stench as we clipped off matted clumps of hair from a sea of necrotic wounds in the dermal layer, connected by a tunnel system of tissue pockets, and crawling with maggots that we picked out with forceps.

That. That was the VA I needed.

The new VA couldn't ever bring herself to show up to any surgical event. Even a mild one. Doesn't make her a bad person. It just wasn't for her.

The manager and I sat her down for a progress discussion one day, less than a month in, and gently laid it out for her. That we appreciated her hard work so far with administrative tasks and cleaning. However, we worried about her in the gore aspect. Did she see herself stepping up to the plate, or did she think veterinary medicine might not be her calling? I already knew it wasn't, but we asked her to go home and think about it, and to let us know her answer the following day.

"Ok," she agreed. "Is it ok if I finish cleaning the kennels before I go home?"

I was admittedly touched by the classy offer.

"That's perfectly fine, if you'd like to."

She did so, then went home. Came to the sensible conclusion, thankfully, and called to let us know the next day.

Most employees that don't work out aren't always so dramatic. But then again …

Another one was a flighty girl whose head was always somewhere else. Terrible work ethic. If I asked her to clean a mess of a kennel, I'd often come in the next day to find she'd done a cursory wipe on the floor of the kennel, but hadn't touched the spray of fecal matter, blood, or saliva that covered the rest of the surfaces. That whole attention to detail thing? Yeah. I need to trust you can accomplish your tasks without me needing to re-do it.

Or I might have taken time to explain something to her, such as how she could prepare lab samples for me, if I was busy elsewhere.

"… and then you'll set the tube here with the coverslip on it. Does that make sense?"

She'd be all smiles and respond with something along the lines of, "Brian did the cutest thing the other day!"

And I'd realize she didn't listen to a damn thing I said, too busy thinking about her friends, and whoever the hell Brian is. I still don't know. She never gave me context before such statements. Just started talking about friends of hers I'd never met or heard of. She didn't last long. Especially after we found out she'd left a few boarding cats locked up in their small hidey-hole cubbies, after cleaning the rest of the kennels. It's only ok to block the entrance to those cubby holes for *a minute* to accomplish your task in the main part of the kennel, if you need the cat out of your way. She wasn't paying attention and left them trapped all night in an enclosed box, nearly suffocating them. Twice.

The last honorable mention was before my time in this particular clinic. There was once an older employee who got busy behind the desk, taking phone calls during a late afternoon. A regular client walked in. Still tied up, she told the client they could go refill their prescription themselves from the medicine shelf. The client was in some kind of medical field, so the employee assumed they'd know what they were looking for.

... They didn't, and unwittingly took home the wrong prescription. A heavy sedative, rather than the needed therapy.

That employee didn't have to be fired. They just stopped showing up, knowing full well their shameful fuck-up.

Rewards & Compassion Fatigue

"… Empathy is a finite resource. You can run out. As a normal, psychological response, you cannot give of yourself again and again and again without replenishing."
—Emmett Fitzgerald

Compassion fatigue is the kind way of saying you're burnt the fuck out.

When the client opens up to you about a devastating situation in their family life, and the family pet—in your care– is the only thing getting them through it? Meanwhile, you feel nothing but numbness as you explain what Scruffy's terminal diagnosis means. Or the fourth client in a week has called, begging you to let their pet be seen today, even though they don't get paid for another two weeks. When it doesn't seem to make you feel that squirming of discomfort in the pit of your stomach anymore. Instead, after you hang up the phone, you check the clock to see how much more time until lunch break …?

That's compassion fatigue.

This apathy zone becomes a battle. How did you get here?

You swung so hard on your emotional pendulum towards the empathy zone, that inevitably, you had to crash hard into the opposite wall. That numbness of feeling. Apathy. When you're too exhausted to feel anything about it, anymore.

There's a lot of filler in-between those polarizing zones, yes. More regulated emotions, appropriate in a given situation. Which doesn't mean it all has to be positive. Sometimes anger, sadness, or frustration are warranted, just as much as joy or contentment. But it needs to be kept in check. We have to safeguard our range of emotions.

We have to take care of ourselves, first.

Instead of pouring so much of ourselves into cases with empathy, what medical professionals have to practice more often is sympathy. For the sake of longevity in a medical field. When one sympathizes, we understand the feelings of another and can express the sentiment appropriately. Meanwhile, when one empathizes, depth is involved. Really *feeling* what the other being is feeling. And that is where veterinary professionals need to be wary. It's inevitable that we'll feel empathy for our patient or client sometimes. It's why we got into the career. None of us started out as the numb apathetic. But it's not sustainable to feel empathy, day in and day out. We wouldn't be able to get out of our beds if we took it all onto our shoulders. Dwelling on every unjust moment, too depressed to move. Unable to stomach the idea of breakfast, let alone getting into our car to drive to work where there will be more sadness waiting for us.

Quite early on in my career, an appointment went awry. My patient crashed in a despondent way I didn't understand, while I was restraining her. The vet took her from me and urged the client to rush his pet to the nearby emergency clinic for more comprehensive care. I didn't sleep that night. Lying there, wide awake, I was sick to my stomach. Trying to discern what I had done wrong. Obsessing over how the frail old owner was going to handle the demise of his beloved dog, Sadie.

The next morning, I had the day off. A rare day of freedom without work or school was a day to be enjoyed. Still, I hadn't moved to get out of bed.

By 8:30 or 9:00 a.m., my phone rang. I saw it was my place of employment. Nervously, I answered. "Hello?"

The vet I'd worked with the night before greeted me by name.

"How are you?" she asked in a deliberate tone.

"Oh … just … lying here," I said lamely.

"I figured. I didn't sleep well, either. But I thought you'd wanna know what came back on Sadie's report."

With a near gasp, I clung to her words. Savoring the explanation of an internal issue that had come to light after extensive diagnostics—which could be medically managed—and had nothing to do with improper restraint. In fact, the vet complimented me, thinking I'd restrained Sadie very well in the circumstance. In short, it wasn't my fault. And Sadie was going to be fine.

I've never forgotten the vet's kind consideration in calling me at home to reassure me about the case. She didn't have to. At the time, I was the lowest rank on the team and could have been easily forgotten. The feelings of guilt and concern for a patient extend to everyone in the hospital, though. We all care.

I worry about the bleeding hearts trying to be a part of this field. I might have been that idealist once. Ready to cure everything and save all the animals. To be honest, I miss a little bit of that side of me. The hopeful optimism. Bitter jadedness seems to creep into my thoughts more frequently, as of late. If there was a way to tell that earlier version of myself to manage expectations, would the burnout be less severe? Or would I have unfairly tempered the sense of passion I felt when I was new to the game? I don't have that answer, but what I do know now is I can't save everything. None of us can. Not individually, nor even as a team. Sometimes we have to accept our limitations. I'm not trying to promote the acceptance of mediocrity or offer excuses to be a lazy fuck. Rather, we have to call it when we're pushed to capacity on caseload. When we've done all we can. When we can't make the client happy. Or when we can't offer charity to those in need.

To learn to sympathize but be cautious at how much we empathize. Our well is not inexhaustible. We can't save everything, but if we can offer quality care to the majority that we *can* help, that's a difference worth making.

Sometimes resources are your limitation. Before finally biting the bullet and buying me a new digital radiograph machine, one employer had held onto his old film processor long after it should have been replaced. When I first started at this practice, the equipment was manageable. Tanks had to be filled with their respective liquids, and hoses turned on to their proper settings. I knew how to shoot the X-ray, take the cassette to the dark room to remove the film, and run it through the dip tanks of the processor. Fixative, developer, and rinse cycles. Elders in the profession will be familiar with the routine.

It was time-consuming, labor-intensive, and not particularly good quality when the finished result finally came out. When it was a newer machine, the films were decent. But after decades of use, it was wearing down. I noticed a significant decline just in the few years since I'd started this job. We'd go through the stress of prepping the equipment, patient handling, and then end up with films that were hardly diagnostic quality anymore. I mean, embarrassing. Near worthless. I used to dread the moments when the veterinarian would make the recommendation for radiographs, secretly hoping the client would decline, just so I wouldn't have to struggle with the process. That's a terrible thought to have, for a test you know is needed.

It all came to a head one day. The rotors were sticking in the tanks, not catching the film to move it through. Despite my best efforts to cleanse the rollers so they'd run smoothly, it wasn't cooperating. The whole device wasn't sitting flat enough and one of the tanks had a perpetual leak. Things just weren't working when I needed to take X-rays of the young doodle that had probably eaten a rope toy.

Given my love and propensity for swearing, no doubt colorful words were said as the doctor came back to check if I was ready for the patient. Seeing my stress, he thought he might sidestep the topic of technical issues. Instead, he tried to soothe me. By reminding me of the client's tragic personal history. How they'd recently lost a child and how devastating it was for them. How this dog belonged to said child. How doggo meant so much to the family.

I knew all that already. It wasn't what I wanted to hear. Rather than an appropriate response to the doctor, what came out of my mouth was less than ideal. Something to the effect of, "Well, I must have a heart of stone, because I don't fucking care right now!"

So, that became the infamous day the doctor broke me. The radiograph processor broke me. The dark-humored joke among my coworkers, that I possessed a black heart. I still get flack for it.

It was a terrible thing to say. No two ways about it. Some of it was frustration in the moment over that damn machine. Some of it was the serious burnout I was feeling about the job. Shutting down in a moment that called for my better nature to rise to compassion. Instead, it wasn't there.

I did soon get the digital radiograph equipment that brought us up to speed with the rest of the world. And caused me far less anguish. Clear pictures with a few clicks and a press of a button. It's been years now, and I still recall the date of its arrival. A lovely anniversary.

I'm not proud of that meltdown, but it's real. Medical professionals have to compartmentalize their emotions, if they're going to be able to continue in their job for a significant length of time. Psychologists would probably tell you this is a defense mechanism to get you through something stressful or traumatic. A means of temporary coping. I'm guessing, anyways. I have zero credentials in psychology, so don't count on me for that.

But that means sometimes I have had to help in that euthanasia exam room, as a family is saying goodbye to their beloved pet. I can sympathize and show the proper professional face of understanding support, maybe offer a gentle hug with a box of tissues, if it's appropriate. We've all been there. We know how hard it is to let go of our companions. But what I can't do is be a sobbing mess alongside them. In fact, I don't consider it appropriate for *me* to be the weepy one. A lump in your throat or a single tear? Sure. We're human. It happens. Even with my black heart. But it's not for me to be the dramatic mourner; it's the client's pet, and it's not about me. I'm there to offer calm and reassurance that this is the right thing for the patient. And because immediately after I leave their exam room, I have to hop into the next one, where the young family is excited about their new puppy. There, my voice must go up five octaves as I squeal in delight over cuteness and buckle down for discussions of vaccine boosters and potty training. Beginnings and endings rolled into packed moments.

Veterinary professionals, I implore you once more. Learn to *sympathize* with an owner but not *empathize* so frequently.

Those cases do happen. The ones where you wonder if you did the right thing. Or if something didn't go well with the procedure, the blame that goes with it. The early incident with Sadie was far from the last time. I've had sleepless nights over a case. But those nights have to be infrequent, otherwise no one would be able to do this.

The veterinary field is starting to realize the levels of compassion fatigue (burnout) we face, and how severely it's impacted a concerning number of those professionals. I'm not going to complain about this awareness being brought into the spotlight. I've felt those emotions. Exhaustion, depression, numbness, and sometimes even hopelessness. I would argue to a lesser degree, it's normal for us to feel that way. Sometimes. But if it's plaguing, I hope with every part of me that my cohorts in the field look for those existing channels of help. Whether they need better coping mechanisms, a refreshing perspective, or if they're even at the point of saying this employment is no longer for them, I hope they do what they need for their own mental health, because their life is more valuable than a job. I hope no one feels defined by a career or title. The three little letters I add after my name on professional correspondence do not define who I am, nor do they have any bearing on my self-worth. "RVT" is something I can be proud of earning once, but it needs to stop there.

I need to be able to go home after a shift and turn off thoughts about cases and clients. I'd argue I need that so I can do a good job the next time they need me.

More recently, I've come across my first VA who was inspired to follow in my footsteps. It wasn't her original plan when she started working with me, but some months into her employment, I must have managed to make my role look appealing. Suddenly, she was applying for a tech program, and got in. Then, I felt more responsible. In a small town, I'm the only RVT in my clinic, and her go-to role model of what it means to be one. She's meeting others now, via her studies and hopefully broadening her horizons, but I'm doing my level best to demonstrate professional integrity to her. A healthy work-life balance, too. Things that are important for self-preservation and endurance, besides the never-ending list of hands-on skills asked of a vet tech. She's still young, bright, and I have high hopes for her own journey. I'm honored to have been both a guide and witness to her start. I hope I'm doing well by her.

I started this career path with passion and excitement. That may be harder to detect in my voice anymore, but I hope I haven't killed it altogether. For anyone wanting to make a career of this, I don't think it's enough to say, "I'm here because I like animals." There needs to be something more that drives you. Why? What, specifically? Promoting animal health? Connecting with the clients? I know technicians that have selected particular areas of focus in their work. One is all about geriatric care of pets, and dignity in their hospice days. She's passionate about having those conversations for maximizing quality of life and knowing when it's time for the harder steps. Another was the go-to girl for exotics cases. Obscure question about a frog or your ball python? She's got you. Others acquired specialist certifications, such as in veterinary ultrasound, behaviorism, or ophthalmology. I once toyed with the idea of furthering my dentistry skill. Yeah, I'm a picker. Anyone who's ever scraped satisfying chunks of dental calculus off a dachshund's teeth knows what I'm talking about. Hell, I can get nerdier. I didn't expect to ever give a shit about it, but I love the laboratory stuff. Microscopy is fun for me. I'd be happy to be your parasitology scanner all day long. I'm nose-blind enough to the offensive odors that I can eat my lunch in the same room as all the fecal samples. (Don't look at me, OSHA officers.) The list of specialized options was short when I was in tech school. Not so anymore. I didn't know it had tripled until my VA showed me the current accepted list from the AVMA. They're probably still adding to it.

Hey, if working in practice isn't for you, but you still want to use your veterinary or vet tech degree? You have options in research or industry. Or zoos. Farming. I'm not qualified to speak on those, but plenty are. Reach out. Find what works for you.

Whether or not you choose something that gets you additional credentials, something needs to bring you joy or satisfaction in the job. A reward for working your ass off. If joy is lacking entirely, it's time to reevaluate.

Do that for yourself.

Epilogue

SOAP Notes was a way to vent, in its infancy. A coping method. After many years as a licensed vet tech, I was burnt out. Compassion running pretty thin, in a place that needed me to show up to work with optimism and a full cup.

Instead, I found solace in writing about the all-too-common ridiculous scenarios encountered by veterinary professionals. An airing of grievances, perhaps. What started out as a few humorous anecdotes quickly turned into longer rants. Then pieces I needed to get off my chest, whether about a tough case or a stressful aspect of the field. A chance to be raw and brutally honest. Good, bad, and ugly. At first, these ramblings were never meant to see the light of day. Alas, one thing led to another and now you're holding the damn book.

At its core, this work was not meant to discourage anyone's interest in the field. While many of these pages reflect my cynical nature and stand-out episodes of absurdity, there were many more moments when I poured my heart and mind into the work, receiving goodness in return. Building bonds with colleagues, meeting honorable animal owners, and of course, cherishing the patients themselves. Work I'm proud I was a part of. Memories I'll never forget.

There was an undercurrent of hope that pet owners, or any

animal lover for that matter, might glean something from these stories. Finding humor, an educational moment, or even awareness of what being an animal caregiver is like, behind the scenes. Something to bridge the gap between us.

Eventually though, I realized that I wrote this memoir as a dedication to my fellow veterinary crew, wherever they practice. No matter which role they fulfill, we've all had our share of mental struggle, physical injury, financial stress, or all manner of heartache. I didn't want to continue to hear of folks I cared about feeling alone or overwhelmed without knowing they have resources. Lifelines to turn to when the burden is too heavy. Boundaries to establish. I wanted to share that sense of camaraderie amongst those professionals who do so much for the animals they've studied, that they sometimes forget vet med can chew you up and spit you back out. We're there, time and again, for the animals and their families. But we have to look out for our people, too. For this author, that meant taking a professional break at this stage of my life. A change of scenery. Currently, on a career path that allows me to continue dabbling in editing medical documentation. I must have a weird obsession with SOAP or something … I still love veterinary medicine, and maybe one day, it will be the right moment to jump back into the pool. That eau-de-anal gland-scented, bloody, hypersalivary, shit-filled pool.

That remains to be seen.

Recommended Reading

Nature Wars: The Incredible Story of How Wildlife Comebacks Turned Backyards into Battlegrounds by Jim Sterba—A book for the ecological scholar, or fans of natural history. I read Sterba's accounts of humans versus the natural world (flora and fauna) as a homework assignment, and it was one hell of an eye-opener. Years later, I still think about it. Safe to say, *Nature Wars* informed at least two chapters in this book.

Why Animals Matter: Animal Consciousness, Animal Welfare, and Human Well-being by Marian Stamp Dawkins—A deep dive into understanding how to discuss the animal experience with logic and reasoning, and why to skip the emotional welfare arguments. It benefits everyone to treat animals well, but Dawkins urges the activist to make themselves more credible.

Fuzz: When Nature Breaks the Law by Mary Roach—I could read anything by Roach. The queen of bringing dark humor to scientifically macabre, and yet, educational subjects. *Fuzz* is another great account of interspecies conflicts (man versus animal).

Animal Husbandry by Laura Zigman—Ok, I admit, this book is kinda-not-really about real animals at all, but it's a wildly funny novel of a woman who, after being devastatingly dumped by an alpha man, copes with an intensive study of her male counterparts through the lens of natural selection.

My Family and Other Animals by Gerald Durrell—A 1930s British family looking for a change decide to move to a Greek island. Told through the eyes of the youngest boy, a precocious wildlife-lover. With a *Swiss Family Robinson* flair, but between descriptions of Gerry's zoo of specimens, I cackled loudly at the antics of the chaotic Durrell family.

All Creatures Great and Small by James Herriot—If you've lived under a rock until now, James Herriot is the godfather of veterinary stories. *All Creatures* is the first book in the series about the Yorkshire-based veterinarian. Quaint, charming, wholesome, and he doesn't swear like me.

Acknowledgements

Holy hell, I wrote a book! You're holding it! I'm still stunned, honestly. But this humble, little ol' vet tech's book didn't happen without a lot of folks believing it could happen first.

To the wonderfully supportive and genuine team from Vine Leaves Press: Jessica Bell, for a stunning cover design and your passion for authors. Melanie Faith, for your confidence in this project and giving the green light to *SOAP Notes*. Amie McCracken, for keeping me on track, your reassurances, and answering my ridiculous publication queries. All of you. Appreciation overflows. Truly. For taking a chance on this amateur and seeing the potential in a rough manuscript that wanted to be a book. It's a dream come true that I got to have my Jo March moment.

To Sterling Hooker (the Great), my developmental editor. Thank you, endlessly, for providing the right amount of encouragement (compliments) to indulge my self-esteem, along with enough of a challenge (kick in the bum) to envision what the book could be. When I was sick of looking at the manuscript, your enthusiasm and ideas invigorated me to tackle it again.

Karen Jones, my copy editor. I extend so much gratitude for your discerning eye for details and polishing the final round of this book. And for enduring my profanity.

Fat Fly Design (John), thank you for making my online presence look respectable. Don't you dare let me forget I owe you scotch for, probably, ever.

Michelle & Allison, my kindred spirits. For commiserating when things were tough. For celebrating when things were good. And Amber, for initial faith and kind words when the manuscript was still in early stages.

Not everyone is blessed with an encouraging family. I hit the jackpot. I owe never-ending gratitude to my brother, Jeff, one of my earliest cheerleaders for the project. For feedback and keeping my voice authentic. He believed *SOAP* could be a real book when my confidence was in the gutter. To my sister, Renee, who was a massive supporter and without any goading, ecstatic enough to volunteer the world's best stick-figure illustrations to the narrative. To my sister, Laurie, who lent her applause, marketing ideas, and though she may not know it yet, will probably be guilted into narrating the audiobook. And to Mama and Daddy, ever proud. Always eager to support. Sorry for the language. You did your best with me, I'm sure. XOXO

For my FIL, Mr. Chuck. Thank you for always supporting the arts, and for being this book's unquestioning and enthusiastic Number One fan.

To Husband—James. The one who was tired of watching me scribble nonsense only for me, buried deep and hidden away from the surface of the world. You issued the challenge: write something to share. Something I know. Not sure this creature took the form you imagined, but you supported it the whole way. Ideas and praise. Calming my fears and irrationalities. Giving a sharp editing eye. Reining in my propensity to vomit every overwhelming detail possible but savoring the well-placed bon mot. And no doubt you were thrilled I found an outlet for diarrhea stories, other than our dinner table. *SOAP Notes* wouldn't have happened without you. James—Making you proud is the best feeling in the world. Love you forever.

Finally, cheers to my fellow veterinary teammates. Those who know me personally, and those working their arses off, everywhere. Veterinarians, receptionists, managers, groomers, vet assistants, veterinary teachers, and of course, my own breed: the vet techs. Forgive me, y'all know I like animals more, but you'll always be my human crowd. Helpers are the best kind. The ones improving quality of life for their patients and their families every day. Every one of you has had wisdom. A story. A contribution. I'm fortunate to carry pieces of you with me forever. Thank you for all you've taught me.

Eternally grateful.

Additional thanks to these references:

Dawkins, Marian Stamp. *Why Animals Matter: Animal Consciousness, Animal Welfare, and Human Well-Being*. New York: Oxford University Press. 2012.

DVM360, "*Younger generations are obsessed with their pets*" by Steve Dale, CABC—www.dvm360.com/view/younger-generations-are-obsessed-with-their-pets

Love A Bull, "*The History of Pit Bulls.*"—https://love-a-bull.org/resources/the-history-of-pit-bulls/

NIH National Library of Medicine, "*Gender and Veterinary Medicine*" by Jeanne Lofstedt, DVM.— https://pmc.ncbi.nlm.nih.gov/articles/PMC340187/

Sterba, Jim. *Nature Wars: The Incredible Story of How Wildlife Comebacks Turned Backyards Into Battlegrounds*. New York: Crown. 2012.

Washington State Association of Veterinary Technicians. *History*—www.wsavt.org/history

www.ingramcontent.com/pod-product-compliance
Ingram Content Group UK Ltd.
Pitfield, Milton Keynes, MK11 3LW, UK
UKHW010009031026
15589UKWH00008B/1546

9 783988 321695